Gonadal Tissue Cryopreservation in Fertility Preservation

Nao Suzuki • Jacques Donnez
Editors

Gonadal Tissue Cryopreservation in Fertility Preservation

Springer

Editors
Nao Suzuki
Department of Obstetrics and Gynecology
St. Marianna University School of Medicine
Kawasaki, Kanagawa
Japan

Jacques Donnez
Societe de Recherche pour l'Inferti
Brussels, Belgium

ISBN 978-4-431-55961-0 ISBN 978-4-431-55963-4 (eBook)
DOI 10.1007/978-4-431-55963-4

Library of Congress Control Number: 2016943199

Printed on acid-free paper

This Springer imprint is published by Springer Nature
The registered company is Springer Japan KK

Preface

In young females, treatment of cancer can cause gonadal dysfunction, loss of fertility, and premature menopause. Cryopreservation of gametes and/or embryos and displacement or shielding of the ovaries during radiation therapy are the standard methods for preserving the fertility of young female cancer patients. In 2004, Professor Donnez reported achievement of the first live birth after ovarian tissue cryopreservation and transplantation. Subsequently, ovarian tissue cryopreservation and transplantation has come to be applied clinically as a new option for fertility preservation. In Europe and the United States, a new field named oncofertility has been established to revitalize the medical approaches to fertility preservation in young cancer patients.

It is anticipated that there will be further progress in fertility preservation techniques for young patients with cancer. Progress in fertility preservation is linked to the improved survivorship of young cancer patients and increases options for patients who wish to preserve their fertility. Development of optimum methods for fertility preservation will allow young cancer patients to concentrate on treating their disease. It is more essential than ever to provide patients who require gonadotoxic therapy with information about the risk of loss of fertility and the techniques that are available for fertility preservation. Accordingly, healthcare providers need to keep up with the latest information on fertility preservation, since rapid progress is occurring in this field. When Professor Donnez reported a successful live birth after transplantation of cryopreserved ovarian tissue, it was a breakthrough for both fertility preservation in young cancer patients and research into reproductive medicine. It is now 12 years since that report, and this book, *Gonadal Tissue Cryopreservation and Fertility*, is being published to provide young cancer patients in Asian countries, where oncofertility has attracted increasing attention in recent years, with the latest information in regard to fertility preservation. I would like to express my deepest gratitude to Professor Donnez, who served as a coeditor of this book. He has been my mentor and has provided willing cooperation during the publication process. I also express my heartfelt thanks to Ms. Makie Kambara and Ms. Kanako Honma at Springer Japan KK, who gave me the precious opportunity to publish this book. I sincerely hope that young cancer patients can beat their disease and that we can achieve a better quality of life for the survivors.

Kawasaki, Kanagawa, Japan Nao Suzuki

Contents

1 **Oocyte Cryopreservation** 1
Javier Domingo, Ana Cobo, and Antonio Pellicer

2 **Controlled Ovarian Stimulation Protocols in Cancer Patients** 21
Hakan Cakmak and Mitchell P. Rosen

3 **Embryo Cryopreservation in Breast Cancer Patients** 39
Giuliano Bedoschi and Kutluk Oktay

4 **Ovarian Tissue Cryopreservation: Slow Freezing** 53
Sonia Herraiz, Cesar Diaz-Garcia, and Antonio Pellicer

5 **Ovarian Tissue Cryopreservation: Ovarian Cortical Tissue Vitrification** 79
Yodo Sugishita, Shu Hashimoto, Takayuki Yamochi, Suguru Igarashi, Mariko Nakajima, Chie Nishijima, Seido Takae, Yuki Horage, Kazuhiro Kawaura, Yoshihiko Hosoi, Yoshiharu Morimoto, and Nao Suzuki

6 **Ovarian Tissue Freezing and Transplantation: Current Status** . . . 95
Jacques Donnez and Marie-Madeleine Dolmans

7 **Heterotopic Ovarian Tissue Transplantation** 105
Michelle Soares, Marie-Madeleine Dolmans, and Jacques Donnez

8 **Sperm Cryopreservation** 125
Takeshi Shin, Mai Fukushima, Akane Miyata, and Hiroshi Okada

9 **Testicular Tissue Cryopreservation** 141
Herman Tournaye, Greta Verheyen, and Ellen Goossens

10 IVA and Ovarian Tissue Cryopreservation 149
Kazuhiro Kawamura

11 Risk of Transferring Malignant Cells with Transplanted Frozen-Thawed Ovarian Tissue 161
Marie-Madeleine Dolmans and Michelle Soares

12 Artificial Ovary 175
Christiani A. Amorim

Chapter 1
Oocyte Cryopreservation

Javier Domingo, Ana Cobo, and Antonio Pellicer

Abstract Fertility preservation has become an emerging discipline for any patient whose reproductive function is threatened. Oocyte vitrification is an established method that provides an excellent clinical outcome. It has become an important part of cancer treatment, but also for other non-oncological reasons, with age or the delay of motherhood as the most frequent reasons nowadays for patients to vitrify their oocytes in order to avoid the age-related infertility. Oocyte vitrification is also useful in different gynecological situations in the clinical practice in assisted reproductive technology (ART) where the delayed embryo transfer should be recommended, such as high risk of hyperstimulation syndrome, bleeding, or the presence of hydrosalpinx or polyps. Clinical pregnancy rates in both cancer and social indications are similar to those observed in conventional IVF treatments, with no increase in adverse obstetric and perinatal outcomes in children conceived from vitrified oocytes or embryos. But there are some limitations that must be known: limited number of IVF cycles depending on the number of vitrified MII oocytes, and survival rates after warming or the outcome of IVF with vitrified oocytes are highly dependent on maternal age at the time of freezing.

Keywords Oocyte • Cryopreservation • Vitrification • Fertility preservation

1.1 Introduction

Oocyte cryopreservation has entailed important advantages for human IVF as advances in cryopreservation methodologies have dramatically improved the efficiency of oocyte cryopreservation in the last few years. Vitrification has proven to

J. Domingo (✉)
IVI Las Palmas, Avda. Juan Carlos I, 17, 35010 Las Palmas de Gran Canaria, Spain
e-mail: javier.domingo@ivi.es

A. Cobo
IVI Valencia, Valencia, Spain

A. Pellicer
University and Polytechnic Hospital La Fe, Valencia, Spain

University Medical School, Valencia, Spain

N. Suzuki, J. Donnez (eds.), *Gonadal Tissue Cryopreservation in Fertility Preservation*, DOI 10.1007/978-4-431-55963-4_1

be a very useful tool for oocyte cryopreservation, becoming a great option for a variety of patients.

Advances in oncological treatments and better screening programs have significantly improved survival rates for young patients suffering from different malignancies [1, 2]. These increasing survival rates have encouraged us to focus on the irreversible consequences of chemotherapy, which become more relevant, and have led to increase the number of patients demanding oocyte vitrification prior to chemotherapy during the last years. However, these procedures should not be limited to patients undergoing cancer therapies, but also applied to any situations where the reproductive function is threatened as some other non-oncological conditions [3], and even more oocyte cryopreservation could meet the expectations of women wishing to delay childbearing for a variety of reasons, simplify the egg donation programs, or just offer a less ethically disputable alternative to embryo cryopreservation [3, 4].

Therefore, since fertility preservation procedures showed benefit for medical or nonmedical patients, a new field in assisted reproductive technology (ART) arose and a new population appeared in fertility clinics.

Moreover, the habitual strategy in assisted reproduction has changed considerably and has given solutions to different clinical situations as unexpected lack of spermatozoa, the presence of polyps or hydrosalpinx during the ovarian stimulation, or high risk of hyperstimulation syndrome in which oocyte cryopreservation can be conducted [5, 6].

Fertility preservation should be considered for oncological patients since the moment the diagnosis is confirmed. At this respect several strategies have been proposed to protect or preserve the ovarian function in patients undergoing chemotherapy [7]. Some of them have demonstrated their efficiency, while others are under evaluation or still need to be improved [8, 9].

Immature egg retrieval for further in vitro maturation (IVM) and vitrification, although of great interest in the future, still does not offer feasible options to the patients [10]. There is no doubt that it will have an important role in the future, as trend on fertility preservation techniques is directed to the combination of ovarian tissue cryopreservation as a source of follicles for further retrieval of immature oocytes and in vitro maturation and later vitrification subsequently, which would make avoidance of the ovarian stimulation or the delay on the initiation of chemotherapy possible.

Oocytes may be cryopreserved at any stage, but mature or germinal vesicle (GV) stage oocytes for later IVM are preferred, although more efficacy has been observed when those GV are matured first with vitrification only for those reaching maturity instead of vitrifying GV and then matured in vitro after warming [10].

1.2 Oocyte Vitrification

Vitrification has nowadays completely replaced the conventional technique of slow freezing, since results observed with this approach are significantly lower, and though it is considered the current method of choice to cryopreserve human oocytes and blastocysts, providing an excellent clinical outcome [11]. Oocyte vitrification is an established method, no longer considered experimental [8] as it keeps developmental competence after warming and has been proven to provide consistent success, with high survival rates and pregnancy and implantation rates similar to those obtained with fresh oocytes [12]. Furthermore, the approach is simple and feasible and, regarding the outcomes achieved, effective and consistent.

Historically, the slow-cooling method for oocyte cryopreservation was hampered due to its low efficiency and because it did not guarantee reproducible results. Nearly 100 frozen eggs were needed to achieve a live birth, demonstrating the difficulty and lack of progress performed. However, in later years, the success rate increased due to a better understanding of oocyte physiology, the use of improved media, and of course the leap came when vitrification was incorporated [13].

Vitrification consists in solidification of a solution by extreme elevation of viscosity using high cooling rates from −15,000 to −30,000 °C/min, avoiding the transition temperature for the crystallization of the solution and preventing the formation of intracellular ice crystals, and thus the damage and the osmotic effects caused by ice formation [14]. The real relevance of the oocyte vitrification approach is that it is able to provide the opportunity of postpone childbearing to whenever the patient wishes, or the time she is cured from the cancer that motivated oocyte vitrification, allowing similar IVF cycle prognosis to the moment of vitrification but a few years later. The developmental capability of embryos obtained from vitrified oocytes is maintained with the use of this technique, with no significant differences observed in fertilization rates, embryo cleavage, or clinical results to those achieved with fresh oocytes [11, 12].

Contribution of vitrification has been high, although there are some potential drawbacks associated, especially with the first protocols applied. One of these problems is the toxicity inherent to the use of cryoprotectants which can be reduced by the use of an adequate combination of cryoprotectants (ethylene glycol + dimethyl sulfoxide (DMSO) + sucrose) [15] or by using very low volumes when loading the samples, increasing considerably the cooling rate and allowing to the reduction of the cryoprotectant concentration used [13].

Several storage systems have been designed. Carriers for loading and storing oocytes, all minimal volume containers, can be "open or closed systems" (open or closed pulled straws, Cryoloop, Cryotop, Cryolock, Hemi-Straw system, Cryolife, CryoTip, Fibre Plug, etc.). Close systems prevent the direct contact with liquid nitrogen, thus avoiding the hypothetical risk of cross-contamination, but greatly slow the cooling rate compromising survival rates as a result. However, it should be mentioned that closed systems provide efficient survival rates and clinical outcomes for early cleavage and blastocyst stage embryos. Anyway, so far the most preferred method for oocyte vitrification is the open system due to its ability to provide highly consistent efficient survival rates and clinical outcomes.

The Cryotop method is a minimal volume device where oocytes are vitrified in volumes lower than 0.1 μl, preserving their capacity for fertilization and further development after warming [13]. In our experience at IVI group with the Cryotop method, survival rates of 97 % have been referred in young patients, with no differences in fecundation and implantation rates, embryo quality, or clinical results when compared to those achieved with fresh oocytes [12, 16]. With this device, the final volume is ten times less than other systems that use minimum volume; therefore freezing rates of –23,000 °C/min are achieved, and moreover, the total concentration of cryoprotectants is reduced to 30 %. Another advantage of the Cryotop method is that it will allow warming rates of 43,000 °C/min, higher to those achieved with other techniques, with ice formation being virtually impossible, which completely eliminates freezing damage and definitely excludes the risk of the zona pellucida being fractured [13].

The risk of cross-contamination has been a point of concern for open systems. Cross-contamination has been related to liquid nitrogen tanks in experimental conditions [17] but never has been reported related to ART cryotransfers. Oocyte cryopreservation procedures have to be efficient and consistent but also safe, and to prevent the risk associated with the direct contact with liquid nitrogen during storage, different strategies have been proposed, as the sterilization of the liquid nitrogen by filtering or by ultraviolet irradiation [18] or the use of vapor phase storage tanks that guarantee optimal conditions during storage at the same temperature of the liquid nitrogen but without being in contact with it and no negative effect on survival and outcome of those vitrified oocytes [19].

Another point of concern about its safety has been the possibility of increasing aneuploidies in the embryos resulting from warmed oocytes, and as a cryopreservation technique, the oocyte vitrification process has to maintain also the structural and genetic integrity. For many years, it has been suggested that the impaired potential of thawed oocytes could be related to the meiotic spindle's high sensitivity to cryopreservation, which may cause an increase in aneuploidy rates affecting the resulting embryos. Different publications showed no abnormal or stray chromosomes from previous frozen oocytes [20] and no differences in the rate of embryonic aneuploidies between embryos from fresh or temporarily vitrified oocytes from the same cohort after microarray analysis [21]. As a result, no significant increase in abnormalities in pregnancies derived from cryostored oocytes has been reported [21, 22]. These results indicate that the chromosome segregation during the anaphase is not impaired by the vitrification process or that it has the capability of restoration. Similar results were found irrespective of different vitrification protocols used, with similar normal spindle configuration between fresh and vitrified oocytes showing that the MII spindle returns to its normal configuration after 3 h of post-thawing incubation under standard conditions [23].

1.3 Technical Aspects of Oocyte Vitrification

The capability of preventing ice formation during all phases of the vitrification process (cooling, exposure to the cryoprotectants, storage, or warming) will condition the feasibility of the oocyte. Crystallization is not compatible with any living organism. There are several factors depending on the oocyte itself that can condition its viability, as its big volume (~150 μm) or its spherical shape, and the content being very rich in water. That gives worse tolerance and hinders the uniform distribution of cryoprotectants, increasing the risk of crystallization. And of course the number of cells is important, and so it can be considered an "all or nothing phenomenon" after warming, as the oocyte is a single cell in comparison with embryos or other tissues.

Another factor that determines the oocyte's viability at cryopreservation is the presence of the meiotic spindle in metaphase II oocytes. Its integrity can be affected by changes of temperature and though the risk of aneuploidies may be increased. Depolymerization of the meiotic spindle occurs at low temperature with tubulin disassembling during the dilution step at warming, although it usually repolymerizes itself after returning to the physiological temperature, reassembling the meiotic spindle. Any deleterious effect of crystallization on the meiotic spindle, which contains the chromosomes aligned, would affect its integrity and consequently its outcome originating aneuploid embryos.

The main potential drawbacks associated with the great cryo-sensibility of oocytes are chilling injury, crystallization, and cryofracture.

Chilling injury mainly associated with slow freezing, may occur at the transition between 15 and –5 °C. This effect on the cells affects the lipids of the membrane and the microtubules of the meiotic spindle and hardens the zona pellucida, being highly vulnerable to low temperatures [24]. This effect can be avoided with a fast transition through this range, with the high cooling rate procedures as provided by vitrification.

Crystallization of the medium surrounding the cells or their cytoplasm is one of the most frequent harmful effects of slow freezing by acting mechanically on the cell structures. During the equilibrium the oocytes respond osmotically to the hypertonic solution of cryoprotectants by means of dehydration. Intracellular ice formation usually occurs when the cell is not sufficiently dehydrated, at the transition between –5 and –80 °C, damaging mechanically the structure of the cell membranes and affecting its viability, especially at thawing [25]. Vitrification is able to virtually avoid crystallization.

Cryofractures affect mainly the zona pellucida, at the range between –50 and –150 °C, due to the mechanical effect of ice crystals [25].

Oocytes suffer an evident shrinkage at dehydration, but gradually re-expand and recover their initial appearance as soon as the cryoprotectant permeates into the cytoplasm. These drastic changes occurring during vitrification may cause subcellular effects on the oocytes. At warming, it's important to avoid variations in the temperature since Cryotops are taken from the storage bank until they are immersed directly into the plate with the devitrification solution. The temperature of the medium is also very important, which has to be at 37 °C to allow warming rates so high as 43.000 °C/min, and then continue with the dilution solution and removal of cryoprotectants and replacement of cellular fluids prior to washing. In conclusion, the speed of both the vitrification and the warming steps is critical, and any variation of temperature will condition the survival of the vitrified oocytes by increasing the risk of ice crystal formation.

1.4 Clinical Aspects of Oocyte Cryopreservation

Fertility preservation started becoming increasingly important to improve the quality of life in cancer survivors. But fertility preservation should not be limited only to cancer patients but in any situation in which ovarian function is compromised, as other non-oncological diseases or different situations related to ovarian surgery as endometriosis, or just simply women who wish to delay childbearing. A variety of techniques are available for fertility preservation, and they can be used individually or together in the same patient to maximize efficiency.

The ovarian cortex incorporates a finite number of primordial follicles, which will decrease with age due to mechanisms of ovulation and especially for atresia. Fertility potential may be compromised in cases of gonadal removal by surgery, as a consequence of the use of chemotherapy, abdominal or pelvic radiation therapy, or even due to the tumor itself acting on the gonads. Radiotherapy and chemotherapy will, therefore, accelerate the natural decline in the number of follicles [26].

Gonadotoxicity, understood as a reduction of ovarian activity, will depend on various factors, such as age; ovarian reserve; type of chemotherapy, especially the use of alkylating agents; type of cancer; and cumulative doses received [27, 28]. As it is an effect directly related to age and the initial state of gonads, young patients may confer some protective effect since many recover their ovarian function and reproductive capability once chemotherapy is completed, especially with low-dose and low-gonadotoxic chemotherapy [29]. But although many may recover their ovarian function after chemotherapy, egg quality may be suboptimal, so the possibility of pregnancy will maintain decreased. Therefore, options to preserve fertility should be considered from the moment of diagnosis.

Most combination chemotherapy regimens include the alkylating agent cyclophosphamide, which is known to cause a significant loss in ovarian follicle reserve, which may result in infertility and early menopause. Radiotherapy and chemotherapy cause irreversible destruction of germ cells by a direct apoptotic effect on oocytes, with a loss of gonadal hormones and increasing the possibility of germ cell mutagenicity and teratogenic effects [30]. The effect of chemotherapy on the ovary is not an all-or-nothing phenomenon, but can be severe or cumulative with the ovaries having limited recovering capability. This impossibility of regeneration after damage produced by cancer treatments, which is progressive and irreversible, and ovarian reserve decreasing with age will mark the ovarian response to chemo- and radiotherapy. Women who have been treated with chemo- or radiotherapy may have irregular periods but also infertility and even premature ovarian failure with decreased follicular pool as a consequence of germinal damage. Thus, cumulative dose in adolescents to cause premature ovarian failure is higher than in adult women [26–28].

In conclusion, chemotherapy and radiotherapy have a major impact on reproductive potential, and fertility preservation procedures should be carried out prior to these treatments. The need for fertility preservation has to be weighed against gonadotoxicity related to the type and doses of the chemotherapy the patient will receive [28] and morbidity and mortality associated with cancer itself.

But oncological treatments are not the only causes that lead to ovarian failure. Nowadays, the most frequent reason why patients decide to vitrify their oocytes for fertility preservation is the delay of motherhood, due to different social and economic factors associated with modern lifestyle. The negative effect of age on fertility is well established, especially in women over 35 years of age, for whom the poorer quality of oocytes and the decreasing ovarian reserve are of great concern as will condition future subfertility [31, 32]. In these cases, cryobanking their own oocytes is a good option for women who plan to delay childbearing.

Several strategies have been proposed for fertility preservation, but two are the main techniques usually proposed to patients: oocyte vitrification and ovarian tissue cryopreservation, although not exclusive, each one with its advantages and limitations.

Ovarian tissue cryopreservation may allow patients to achieve pregnancies spontaneously without limitation in time while the graft is viable and incidentally bring the woman some hormonal levels in the event of total loss of ovarian function. Although live births are increasing constantly with this technique, its true effectiveness is discussed as the total number of failed implants is not well known. This reason along with the possibility of reseeding tumor cells into cured patients with the graft makes still considered investigational [33].

Oocyte vitrification should be the elective approach for patients demanding fertility preservation for nonmedical reasons. Oocyte vitrification is an established method no longer considered experimental, with consistent results and whose efficiency has been proven as previously commented, but has its own limitations, as the number of available metaphase II oocytes which can limit the number of IVF attempts and survival rates, mainly related to patient's age and quality of eggs, and more vitrified oocytes are required to achieve equivalent cumulative ongoing pregnancy rates in blastocysts than when early cleavage-stage embryos are transferred [34].

Specialists, patients, and their families should be aware that fertility preservation can be considered and reproductive function preserved in any condition where fertility can be threatened. A multidisciplinary collaboration in the management of these patients between oncologists, gynecologists, surgeons, hematologists, pediatricians, and reproductive specialists is needed to improve awareness and availability. Decisions should be made individually, both when recommending fertility preservation or allow attempting a pregnancy.

1.4.1 Clinical Indications

The usefulness of this strategy becomes very clear for those women who need an option for fertility preservation, like patients diagnosed with malignant diseases receiving chemo or radiotherapy and that will suffer from gonadal failure and infertility after their cancer treatment or other non-oncological conditions such as autoimmune disorders that need to be treated with chemotherapy. Women who postpone conception until late reproductive years, recurrent endometriosis, or some chromosomal abnormalities that can lead to ovarian failure can also benefit of this fertility preservation procedure [3, 8, 35].

Cryopreservation of the female gametes has represented an important challenge since the beginning of ART given its potential for overcoming several of the problems that arise during fertility treatment, such as people with high risk of hyperstimulation syndrome, appearance of an hydrosalpinx or polyps during the stimulation, unexpected absence of spermatozoa the day of the ovum pickup, low-responder patients to accumulate oocytes from two or three stimulation cycles, any bleeding prior to embryo transfer, and ethical concern about embryo cryopreservation [36, 37]. Moreover, the establishment of egg banking system for ovum donation programs would considerably simplify the logistics by which oocytes could be donated since no synchronization between the donor and recipient should be needed, shortening the days of estradiol replacement until donation. Oocyte cryopreservation, similarly to semen banks, would also allow a more accurate screening for viral infections [38].

When planning oocyte cryopreservation for fertility preservation in a cancer patient, always under our criteria with the oncologist's authorization, different factors must be considered, as age, time until chemotherapy will begin, the need of an ovarian stimulation, and whether the tumor is hormone sensitive or not. For those cases where the time hiatus between diagnosis and treatment is not always available or the potential risks associated with high estrogen levels do not recommend an ovarian stimulation, or in the case of girls, ovarian tissue cryopreservation for later autotransplantation should be the first elective approach.

Fertility preservation procedures are not limited to cancer patients but can be applied in other non-oncological situations which may lead to ovarian failure, some of them being medical situations while others nonmedical.

Severe systemic autoimmune diseases should be one of these situations as they may require therapy potentially harmful to their ovaries as cyclophosphamide for refractory rheumatoid arthritis [39], for severe manifestations of systemic lupus erythematosus, such as proliferative nephritis, affection of the central nervous system, pneumonitis or severe thrombocytopenia [40], or in other diseases such as Wegener's granulomatosis [41]. Patients needing bone marrow transplantation are also associated with high risk of ovarian failure as high doses of chemo- and radiotherapy are applied to destroy the preexisting bone marrow [42].

Repetitive conservative surgery on the ovaries can also lead to premature ovarian failure by diminishing ovarian reserve, and furthermore the pregnancy rate is almost half the rate obtained after primary surgery [43]. Endometriosis plays an important role as one of the most frequent pathologies in gynecologic surgery, although there are other benign surgical procedures that can result in a loss of ovarian function. Excision of endometriotic cysts is associated with a significant reduction in ovarian reserve as normal ovarian tissue is removed and destructed by electrocoagulation, and therefore they only should be removed if pain, infertility, and large size of the endometriomas obstruct the oocyte retrieval at the ovum pickup [44].

In the same manner, patients with mosaic Turner syndrome should be candidates for oocyte vitrification as premature ovarian failure is commonly associated with this chromosomal abnormality [45] or patients with conservative surgery diagnosed with early-stage borderline ovarian tumors as a preventative measure in case of recurrence and adnexectomy [46].

Ovarian hyperstimulation syndrome (OHSS) is one of the most serious iatrogenic complications of IVF, and embryo transfer should never be done in the same cycle in patients at high risk of it, and therefore an effective strategy could be to vitrify the oocytes for a later embryo transfer in another cycle [47]. In oncological patients cryopreserving their oocytes, many of them young and with good ovarian reserve and whose goal is not to get pregnant, it would be advisable to use protocols with gonadotrophin-releasing hormone (GnRH) antagonists and trigger ovulation with a bolus of GnRH agonist to avoid the possibility of causing OHSS [37]. After GnRH agonist triggering, the antagonist is moved and the receptor is directly activated causing the *flare up* effect which is accompanied by the release of gonadotropins [6]. This *flare up* effect is effective in the final oocyte maturation and ovulation. Advantages consist of the possibility to recover a higher number of mature oocytes [48], shortening of the luteal phase, and avoiding the discomfort related to ovarian hyperstimulation at the time OHSS is largely prevented. This is very important if we consider that most of these patients will start chemotherapy immediately after finishing the process. This should be extended to all patients who wish to vitrify their eggs. Recent publications have reported that this agonist trigger and freeze-all strategy does not prevent severe OHSS at all, as some cases have arisen, so this complication has not been completely eliminated with this approach [49, 50].

Accumulation of oocytes from several ovarian stimulation cycles is a valid strategy for low-responder patients, in order to increase the availability of oocytes to reach a similar situation to normoresponders for a further IVF cycle or if preimplantation genetic screening (PGS) is pretended [51]. This approach is associated with a lower drop-out rate, fewer transfer cancelations, higher live birth rate per intention-to-treat patient, more cycles with vitrified embryos, and higher cumulative pregnancy rate, which endorses the treatment as a successful alternative for low-responder patients. Similar outcome was observed among patients over 40 years of age [52].

Social fertility preservation is a new medical and social phenomenon to prevent age-related subfertility, motivated primarily by the search for a social and labor stability or the absence of a stable partner. The patient vitrifies her oocytes with no medical indication for postponement of childbearing, which means a medical intervention which is not associated with a need. They are fertile and healthy women who choose to delay childbearing for various reasons.

There may be an idea of social fertility preservation postponing the first pregnancy with important demographic and economic consequences related to an inverted population pyramid. The age for a first pregnancy has risen nowadays a mean of 2 years over the past 10 years. Regarding this, the mean age for a first pregnancy in our country has increased to 32 years of age [53]. Age is directly related to subfertility, and nowadays the number of patients in the 40s attempting IVF, with dramatically decreased pregnancy rates, is increasing constantly, some of them with the false idea of ART compensating the natural decline of fertility and taking the success of IVF for granted. More than 50 % of the IVF cycles in Europe are done nowadays in patients over 35 years of age [54]. Oocyte vitrification could be a solution for these patients, even more if there is a family history of premature menopause, so this approach should be not so questioned as it was a few years ago, as it would be useful to prevent infertility related to age [55]. Treating older women with their own young oocytes would help to reach better reproductive outcome and diminish the need of egg donation. Female fertility consistently decreases after the middle of the third decade [56], so oocyte cryopreservation should be done ideally earlier.

Oocyte cryopreservation also will be useful to overcome ethical concerns and legal restrictions in several countries associated with embryo cryopreservation.

1.4.2 Clinical Results and Obstetric Outcome: Limitations of the Procedure

The available knowledge of oocytes from ovum donation programs and also on the autologous IVF cycles carried out with vitrified oocytes offer better outcomes in terms of oocyte survival and embryological development of the vitrified and warmed oocyte in comparison with the slow-freezing procedure and similar clinical results when compared with fresh oocytes [11, 57, 58].

In our experience the developmental capability of embryos obtained from vitrified oocytes is not affected by the vitrification procedure, since fertilization, embryo cleavage, quality, and clinical results are similar to those achieved with fresh oocytes [12]. Survival rates so high as 97 % have been referred for young donor patients [12].

The number of pregnancies resulting after an oocyte cryopreservation process is growing constantly, with no apparent increase in adverse obstetric and perinatal outcomes in children conceived with vitrified oocytes as low birth weight or congenital abnormalities [59, 60]. The incidence of other complications including anemia, diabetes, pregnancy-induced hypertension, preterm premature rupture of membranes, and preterm birth rates is comparable to those observed with fresh oocytes [60].

The availability of egg banking for both ovum donation programs and own oocytes for autologous IVF cycles has proven highly efficient and has conferred remarkable advantages. Outcomes of ongoing data from clinical use of vitrified donor oocytes have confirmed that these procedures are efficient, reliable, safe, and consistent. Cryobanking eggs provides the possibility to match a donor for a recipient from a large donor pool without waiting long for an appropriate match, and donors can carry out their donation cycle independently on the recipient, with no adverse effect on results.

The limitation of the procedure can be given by the number of vitrified MII oocytes that will limit the number of IVF attempts in the future and consequently the availability of embryos and the possibilities of achieving a pregnancy. Age again may condition the results as survival rates decrease with it. Survival of the oocytes is related to the quality of the oocyte what is an age-dependent factor. This lack of survival may serve as a selection filter but overshadows the benefits the procedure could have on low responders, most of them around the 40s. Patients should be advised to ensure a reasonable number of cryopreserved oocytes for which more than one stimulation cycle should be required. The outcome of IVF with vitrified oocytes is, just as for fresh oocytes, highly dependent on maternal age at the time of freezing, but not related to the vitrification process itself [52, 61].

To face the fact of low survival rates in patients where bad oocyte quality may be suspected, embryo cryopreservation instead of oocyte vitrification for differed embryo transfer or just to accumulate for later PGS could be an option as survival rates for them seem to be higher.

Despite oocyte vitrification protocols being simple to perform, experienced hands are needed to guarantee success. A learning curve is necessary to avoid changes in temperature during cooling and warming and results may be influenced until high efficiency is reached.

1.4.3 Ovarian Stimulation

One of the concerns on oocyte cryopreservation is that a prior multiple follicular stimulation is needed as well as a time frame of 2 or 3 weeks, which would delay the beginning of chemotherapy. However, the elapsed time between cancer diagnoses and initiation of treatment may vary among malignancies, especially in breast cancer patients and some leukemias or lymphomas which have to wait 4 or 6 weeks to start the chemotherapy. Another point of concern is whether the stimulation with gonadotropins would affect the evolution of breast cancer, which is the most common malignancy in reproductive age and the most frequent diagnosis of people undergoing any fertility preservation option [62]. High estradiol levels are the main objection for patients with hormone-dependent tumors, as in vitro cellular proliferation has been demonstrated when acute exposure to estrogens occurs, and would contribute to the activation of pro-oncogenes in breast cancer [63, 64]. Recent studies show that exposure to FSH, luteinizing hormone (LH), or human chorionic gonadotropin (hCG) does not appear to cause an increase in cell proliferation in either normal or malignant mammary epithelial cell lines, and so, the potential risk for mammary cell transformation associated with these agents may be related to indirect endocrine effects on breast cell physiology [65].

Patients with hormone-sensitive tumors can benefit from specific protocols with letrozole and FSH proposed to minimize estrogen exposure, resulting in comparable yield of oocyte, and similar estradiol levels with respect to natural cycle in breast cancer patients, with similar recurrence rate to unstimulated breast cancer patients [66, 67]. Tamoxifen has also been proposed as ovarian inductor.

Letrozole is an aromatase inhibitor that has been shown to be effective as ovulation inductor and to reduce the negative feedback that estradiol exerts in the hypothalamus and pituitary resulting in an increased FSH sensitivity of the receptors in the ovarian granulosa cells [68]. As a result, it induces suppression of circulating estradiol levels. In non-hormone-dependent (HD) cancers, COH may be performed using FSH under a habitual GnRH antagonist protocol. In HD cancer patients, letrozole (5 mg/day) is recommended for ovarian stimulation in association to FSH, also under a GnRH antagonist protocol to trigger with a GnRH bolus [69].

An important factor to consider when planning an oocyte vitrification process in an oncology patient is the time available until the start of their cancer treatment. Frequently, one of the most frequent problems we face is that patients are not in the initial follicular phase when they come to start the ovarian stimulation, with risk of delaying even more the corresponding oncological treatment if we wait longer, probably with no time available.

Consequently, the new emergency fertility preservation protocols arise, with stimulation starting at any moment of the cycle unlike conventional stimulation protocols, based on the latest idea that there are several waves of follicular recruitment during the cycle. Starting ovarian stimulation in late follicular or luteal phase would minimize delays and allow more patients to undergo fertility preservation and still proceed with cancer treatment within 2–3 weeks. Luteal phase ovarian stimulation is feasible for producing competent oocytes/embryos in women undergoing IVF/ICSI treatments, with optimal pregnancy outcomes after embryo transfer [70, 71].

The number of oocytes, mature oocytes, and fecundation rate observed within these emergency protocols are similar to those achieved with the habitual protocols starting at the beginning of the cycle, like clinical pregnancy rates, ongoing pregnancy rates, and implantation rates, so this type of stimulation can be very useful for those patients in which time can be decisive. Follicular development and increase of estradiol levels are also similar, even if letrozole is used in breast cancer patients. The length of the stimulation is similar when starting independently in late follicular or luteal phase, but significantly longer than the conventional stimulations, and therefore higher doses of gonadotrophins [70, 71].

1.5 IVI's Fertility Preservation Program: Our Experience

A program for fertility preservation was developed at IVI with the intention to present the current situation of fertility preservation techniques to patients and specialists, offering to all acceptable oncology patients wishing to do it the possibility to vitrify their oocytes prior to chemotherapy treatment.

Although it started in oncological patients, nowadays the main reason for vitrification is age-related or delayed motherhood (65 %) followed by oncological (30 %) and non-oncological (5 %) causes, mostly endometriosis [72].

Social FP cycles have increased exponentially in recent years, with more than 600 cycles performed during the year 2014 throughout the IVI group whereas only 100 cycles due to oncological diagnose. Evolution of the number of oocyte vitrification procedures during the past years for social, non-oncological, and oncological fertility preservation can be seen in Fig. 1.1. Nowadays, one of four cycles is due to fertility preservation at IVI and one of five cycles to social fertility preservation (Fig. 1.2).

Patients who merely vitrify their oocytes to delay childbearing are usually women between 35 and 39 years of age, mostly with a university degree and without a steady partner, with a job and economical independency, and with other priorities in their life at that time. In 2014, 80.7 % of patients were between 35 and 41 years of age, with an average age of 38 years at the moment of

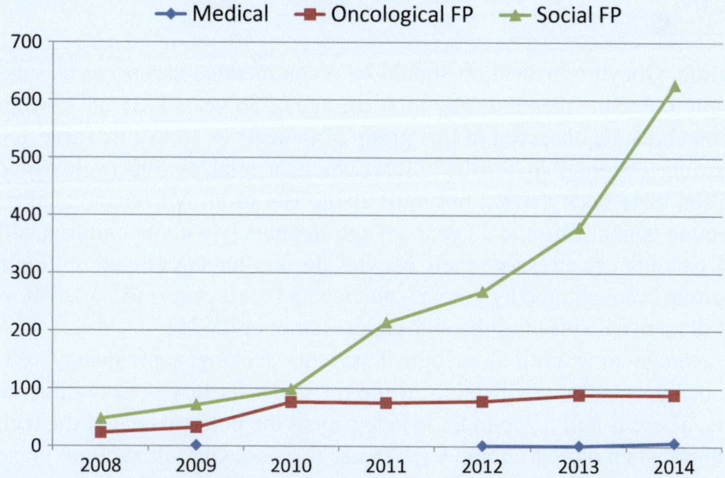

Fig. 1.1 Evolution of the number of oocyte vitrification procedures for social, medical (non-oncological) and oncological fertility preservation (*FP*) along the years

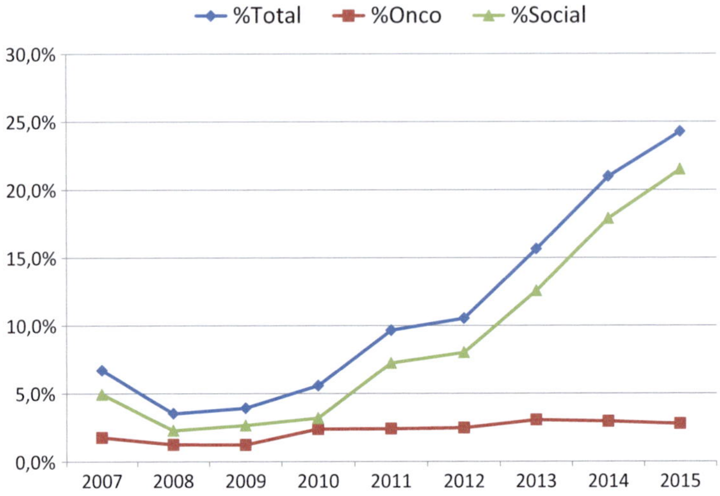

Fig. 1.2 Evolution of the percentage of all vitrification cycles at IVI which are due to oncological and social reasons along the years

Table 1.1 Clinical results observed in social fertility preservation patients seeking a pregnancy that warmed their oocytes

Age	Number procedures	Number patients	Survival rate	Pregnancy rate	Ongoing pregnancy rate	Implantation rate
≤29	7	4	87.8	57.1	57.1	58.3
30–34	19	16	90.9	58.8	52.9	48
35–39	121	78	80	43.9	25.2	30.5
40–44	28	24	85.3	20	13.3	17.4
Total	**175**	**122**	**86**	**43.8**	**28.8**	**32.6**

vitrification. Oocyte vitrification should be recommended earlier, as success rates may begin to decline meaningfully after the age of 36 years [73] and corroborated with clinical results observed in this group of patients as shown in Table 1.1.

Regarding oncological fertility preservation, a total of 595 cycles of oocyte vitrification have been carried out until 2014. The profile of oncological patients is of a young woman, around 32 years of age and mostly without children, although 11 % of patients cryopreserve their oocytes despite having already children. The largest group is constituted by young women with breast cancer (65 %), followed by patients diagnosed with other hematological tumors [72, 74].

The average time until oncological patients seeking a pregnancy use these oocytes is 3 years after vitrification, while for social fertility preservation patients, 2.2 years. There is still a gap in knowledge about the performance of the technique in the future when patients come back to use their oocytes, although at present we have already warmed oocytes corresponding to 25 patients seeking for a pregnancy, with a total of 32 fresh or frozen embryo transfers. Currently 11 pregnancies have

Table 1.2 Clinical results observed in oncological fertility preservation patients seeking a pregnancy that warmed their oocytes

Age	Number procedures	Number patients	Survival rate	Pregnancy rate	Ongoing pregnancy rate	Implantation rate
≤29	2	2	78.6			0
30–34	15	10	85.7	41.7	33.3	26.1
35–39	13	11	78.8	46.1	30.7	28.6
40–44	2	2	94.4			0
Total	**32**	**122**	**86**	**40.74**	**28.8**	**25.5**

been achieved, biochemical excluded, consisting in five living births, three ongoing pregnancies at the moment (one of them being twins), and three clinical abortions. At the moment six patients still have 12 frozen embryos; thus a number of pregnancies may still be increased. Survival rate of 83 %, clinical pregnancy rate of 40.7 %, and ongoing pregnancy rate of 29.6 % with implantation rate of 25.5 % have been observed (Table 1.2).

Despite guidelines suggesting that discussion of fertility preservation should be done prior to starting cancer therapies, it seems to be a lack of implementation in this area, as the number of new cases done every year increases very slowly (Fig. 1.1). It may be due to oncologists directing their patients to the reproduction department of their own hospitals that may be already conducting this technique. Anyway, the increase in the number of cycles is not as pronounced as social fertility preservation.

References

1. Surveillance, Epidemiology and End Results Program, 1975–2003, Division of Cancer Control and Population Sciences, National Cancer Institute, 2006
2. http://www.uv.es/rnti/cifrasCancer.html
3. Domingo J, Cobo A, Sánchez M et al (2011) Principles and practice of fertility preservation. In: Donnez, Kim (eds) Principles and practice of fertility preservation. Cambridge University Press, New York, pp 23–34
4. Cobo A, Domingo J, Pérez S et al (2008) Vitrification: an effective new approach to oocyte banking and preserving fertility in cancer patients. Clin Transl Oncol 10:268–273
5. Jeruss JS, Woodruff TK (2009) Preservation of fertility in patients with cancer. N Engl J Med 360:902–911. doi:10.1056/NEJMra0801454
6. Humaidan P, Kol S, Papanikolaou EG (2011) GnRH agonist for triggering of final oocyte maturation: time for a change of practice? Hum Reprod Update 17:510–524. doi:10.1093/humupd/dmr008
7. Ethics Committee of the American Society for Reproductive Medicine (2005) Fertility preservation and reproduction in cancer patients. Fertil Steril 83:1622–1628
8. The Practice Committees of the ASRM and SART (2013) Mature oocyte cryopreservation: a guideline. Fertil Steril 99:37–43. doi:10.1016/j.fertnstert.2012.09.028

9. Dolmans MM, Luyckx V, Donnez J et al (2013) Risk of transferring malignant cells with transplanted frozen thawed ovarian tissue. Fertil Steril 99:1514–1522. doi:10.1016/j.fertnstert.2013.03.027
10. Cao Y, Xing Q, Zhang ZG et al (2009) Cryopreservation of immature and in vitro matured oocytes by vitrification. Reprod Biomed Online 19:369–373
11. Cobo A, Diaz C (2011) Clinical application of oocyte vitrification: a systematic review and meta-analysis of randomized controlled trials. Fertil Steril 96:277–285. doi:10.1016/j.fertnstert.2011.06.030
12. Cobo A, Kuwayama M, Pérez S et al (2008) Comparison of concomitant outcome achieved with fresh and cryopreserved oocytes vitrified by the Cryotop method. Fertil Steril 89:1657–1664
13. Kuwayama M, Vajta G, Kato O et al (2005) Highly efficient vitrification method for cryopreservation of human oocytes. Reprod Biomed Online 11:300–308
14. Tao T, del Valle A (2008) Human oocyte and ovarian tissue cryopreservation and its application. J Assist Reprod Genet 25:287–296. doi:10.1007/s10815-008-9236-z
15. Vajta G, Nagy ZP (2006) Are programmable freezers still needed in the embryo laboratory? Review on vitrification. Reprod Biomed Online 12:779–796
16. Cobo A, Meseguer M, Remohí J et al (2010) Use of cryo-banked oocytes in an ovum donation programme: a prospective, randomized, controlled, clinical trial. Hum Reprod 25:2239–2246. doi:10.1093/humrep/deq146
17. Bielanski A, Nadin-Davis S, Sapp T et al (2000) Viral contamination of embryos cryopreserved in liquid nitrogen. Cryobiology 40:110–116
18. Parmegiani L, Accorsi A, Cognigni GE et al (2010) Sterilization of liquid nitrogen with ultraviolet irradiation for safe vitrification of human oocytes or embryos. Fertil Steril 94:1525–1528. doi:10.1016/j.fertnstert.2009.05.089
19. Cobo A, Romero JL, Perez S et al (2010) Storage of human oocytes in the vapor phase of nitrogen. Fertil Steril 94:1903–1907. doi:10.1016/j.fertnstert.2009.10.042
20. Boiso I, Marti M, Santalo J et al (2002) A confocal microscopy analysis of the spindle and chromosome configurations of human oocytes cryopreserved at the germinal vesicle and metaphase II stage. Hum Reprod 17:1885–1891
21. Forman EJ, Li X, Ferry KM et al (2012) Oocyte vitrification does not increase the risk of embryonic aneuploidy or diminish the implantation potential of blastocysts created after ICSI: a novel, paired randomized controlled trial using DNA fingerprinting. Fertil Steril 98:644–649. doi:10.1016/j.fertnstert.2012.04.028
22. Cobo A, Rubio C, Gerli S et al (2001) Use of fluorescence in situ hybridization to assess the chromosomal status of embryos obtained from cryopreserved oocytes. Fertil Steril 75:354–360
23. Cobo A, Pérez S, De los Santos MJ et al (2008) Effect of different cryopreservation protocols on the metaphase II spindle in human oocytes. Reprod Biomed Online 173:350–359
24. Vajta G, Kuwayama M (2006) Improving cryopreservation systems. Theriogenology 65:236–244
25. Liebermann J, Dietl J, Vanderzwalmen P et al (2003) Recent developments in human oocyte, embryo and blastocyst vitrification: where are we now? Reprod Biomed Online 7:623–633
26. Larsen EC, Muller J, Schmiegelow K et al (2003) Reduced ovarian function in a long-term survivors of radiation and chemotherapy-treated childhood cancer. J Clin Endocrinol Metab 88:5307–5314
27. Meirow D, Nugent D (2001) The effects of radiotherapy and chemotherapy on female reproduction. Hum Reprod Update 7:535–543
28. Poniatowski BC, Grimm P, Cohen G (2001) Chemotherapy-induced menopause: a literature review. Cancer Invest 19:641–648
29. Brydoy M, Fossa SD, Dahl O et al (2007) Gonadal dysfunction and fertility problems in cancer survivors. Acta Oncol 46:480–489

30. Meirow D, Epstein M, Lewis H et al (2001) Administration of cyclophosphamide at different stages of follicular maturation in mice: effects on reproductive performance and fetal malformations. Hum Reprod 16:632–637
31. Bromer JG, Patrizio P (2008) Preservation and postponement of female fertility. Placenta 29 (Suppl B):200–205. doi:10.1016/j.placenta.2008.07.005
32. Dupas C, Christin-Maitre S (2008) What are the factors affecting fertility in 2008? Ann Endocrinol 69(Suppl 1):S57–S61. doi:10.1016/S0003-4266(08)73970-2
33. Donnez J, Dolmans MM (2015) Ovarian tissue freezing: current status. Curr Opin Obstet Gynecol 27:222–230. doi:10.1097/GCO.0000000000000171
34. Cobo A (2012) Oocyte vitrification: a watershed in ART. Fertil Steril 98:600–601. doi:10.1016/j.fertnstert.2012.07.1096
35. Donnez J (2013) Introduction: fertility preservation, from cancer to benign disease to social reasons: the challenge of the present decade. Fertil Steril 99:1467–1468. doi:10.1016/j.fertnstert.2013.03.040
36. Cobo A, Bellver J, Domingo J et al (2008) New options in assisted reproduction technology: the Cryotop method of oocyte vitrification. Reprod Biomed Online 17:68–72
37. Bodri D, Guillén JJ, Trullenque M et al (2010) Early ovarian hyperstimulation syndrome is completely prevented by gonadotropin releasing-hormone agonist triggering in high-risk oocyte donor cycles: a prospective, luteal-phase follow-up study. Fertil Steril 93:2418–2420. doi:10.1016/j.fertnstert.2009.08.036
38. Cobo A, Remohí J, Chang CC et al (2011) Oocyte cryopreservation for donor egg banking. Reprod Biomed Online 23:341–346. doi:10.1016/j.rbmo.2011.05.014
39. Bernatsky S, Clarke A, Suissa S (2008) Hematologic malignant neoplasms after drug exposure in rheumatoid arthritis. Arch Intern Med 168:378–381. doi:10.1001/archinternmed.2007.107
40. Schroeder JO, Euler H, Loffler H (1987) Synchronization of plasmapheresis and pulse cyclophosphamide in severe systemic lupus erythematosus. Ann Intern Med 107:344–346
41. Langford C (2003) Wegener's granulomatosis: current and upcoming therapies. Arthritis Res Ther 5:180–191
42. Rauck AM, Grouas AC (1999) Bone marrow transplantation in adolescents. Adolesc Med 10:445–449
43. Berlanda N, Vercellini P, Fedele L (2010) The outcomes of repeat surgery for recurrent symptomatic endometriosis. Curr Opin Obstet Gynecol 22:320–325. doi:10.1097/GCO.0b013e32833bea15
44. García-Velasco JA, Somigliana E (2009) Management of endometriomas in women requiring IVF: to touch or not to touch. Hum Reprod 24:496–501. doi:10.1093/humrep/den398
45. Lau NM, Huang JY, MacDonald S et al (2009) Feasibility of fertility preservation in young females with Turner syndrome. Reprod Biomed Online 18:290–295
46. Faluyi O, Mackean M, Gourley C et al (2010) Interventions for the treatment of borderline ovarian tumours. Cochrane Database Syst Rev 8:CD007696. doi:10.1002/14651858.CD007696.pub2
47. Herrero L, Pareja S, Aragonés M et al (2014) Oocyte versus embryo vitrification for delayed embryo transfer: an observational study. Reprod Biomed Online 29:567–572. doi:10.1016/j.rbmo.2014.07.016
48. Humaidan P, Bredkjaer HE, Bungum L et al (2005) GnRH agonist (buserelin) or hCG for ovulation induction in GnRH antagonist IVF/ICSI cycles: a prospective randomized study. Hum Reprod 20:1213–1220
49. Gurbuz AS, Gode F, Ozcimen N et al (2014) Gonadotrophin-releasing hormone agonist trigger and freeze-all strategy does not prevent severe ovarian hyperstimulation syndrome: a report of three cases. Reprod Biomed Online 29:541–544. doi:10.1016/j.rbmo.2014.07.022
50. Santos-Ribeiro S, Polyzos NP, Stouffs K et al (2015) Ovarian hyperstimulation syndrome after gonadotropin-releasing hormone agonist triggering and "freeze-all": in-depth analysis of genetic predisposition. J Assist Reprod Genet 32(7):1063–1068. doi: 10.1007/s10815-015-0498-y

51. Milán M, Cobo AC, Rodrigo L et al (2010) Redefining advanced maternal age as an indication for preimplantation genetic screening. Reprod Biomed Online 21:649–657. doi:10.1016/j.rbmo.2010.06.020
52. Cobo A, Garrido N, Crespo J et al (2012) Accumulation of oocytes: a new strategy for managing low-responder patients. Reprod Biomed Online 24:424–432. doi:10.1016/j.rbmo.2011.12.012
53. http://www.ine.es/daco/daco42/idb/idb.htm
54. Nyboe Andersen A, Goossens V, Bhattacharya S et al (2009) Assisted reproductive technology and intrauterine inseminations in Europe, 2005: results generated from European registers by ESHRE: ESHRE. The European IVF Monitoring Programme (EIM), for the European Society of Human Reproduction and Embryology. Hum Reprod 24:1267–1287. doi:10.1093/humrep/dep035
55. ESHRE Task Force on Ethics and Law, Dondorp W, deWert G et al (2012) Oocyte cryopreservation for age-related fertility loss. Hum Reprod 27:1231–1237. doi:10.1093/humrep/des029
56. Stoop D, Cobo A, Silber S (2014) Fertility preservation for age-related fertility decline. Lancet 384:1311–1319. doi:10.1016/S0140-6736(14)61261-7
57. Edgar DH, Gook DA (2012) A critical appraisal of cryopreservation (slow cooling versus vitrification) of human oocytes and embryos. Hum Reprod Update 18:536–554. doi:10.1093/humupd/dms016
58. Rienzi L, Romano S, Albricci L et al (2010) Embryo development of fresh vs vitrified metaphase II oocytes after ICSI: a prospective randomized sibling-oocyte study. Hum Reprod 25:66–73. doi:10.1093/humrep/dep346
59. Levi PE, Albani E, Morenghi E et al (2013) Comparative analysis of fetal and neonatal outcomes of pregnancies from fresh and cryopreserved/thawed oocytes in the same group of patients. Fertil Steril 100:396–401. doi:10.1016/j.fertnstert.2013.03.038
60. Cobo A, Serra V, Garrido N et al (2014) Obstetric and perinatal outcome of babies born from vitrified oocytes. Fertil Steril 102:1006–1015. doi:10.1016/j.fertnstert.2014.06.019
61. Rienzi L, Cobo A, Paffoni A et al (2012) Consistent and predictable delivery rates after oocyte vitrification: an observational longitudinal cohort multicentric study. Hum Reprod 17:1606–1612. doi:10.1093/humrep/des088
62. Sonmezer M, Oktay K (2006) Fertility preservation in young women undergoing breast cancer therapy. Oncologist 11:422–434
63. Platet N, Cathiard AM, Gleizes M et al (2004) Estrogens and their receptors in breast cancer progression: a dual role in cancer proliferation and invasion. Crit Rev Oncol Hematol 51:55–67
64. Butt AJ, Caldon CE, McNeil CM et al (2008) Cell cycle machinery: links with genesis and treatment of breast cancer. Adv Exp Med Biol 630:189–205
65. Boukaidi SA, Cooley A, Hardy A et al (2012) Impact of infertility regimens on breast cancer cells: follicle-stimulating hormone and luteinizing hormone lack a direct effect on breast cell proliferation in vitro. Fertil Steril 97:440–444. doi:10.1016/j.fertnstert.2011.11.020
66. Oktay K, Hourvitz A, Sahin G et al (2006) Letrozole reduces estrogen and gonadotropin exposure in women with breast cancer undergoing ovarian stimulation before chemotherapy. J Clin Endocrinol Metab 91:3885–3890
67. Azim AA, Costantini-Ferrando M, Oktay K (2008) Safety of fertility preservation by ovarian stimulation with letrozole and gonadotropins in patients with breast cancer: a prospective controlled study. J Clin Oncol 26:2630–2635. doi:10.1200/JCO.2007.14.8700
68. GarcíaVelasco JA, Moreno L, Pacheco A et al (2005) Aromatase inhibitor letrozole increases the concentration of intraovarian androgens and improves in vitro fertilization outcome in low responder patients: a pilot study. Fertil Steril 84:82–87
69. Domingo J, Guillén V, Ayllón Y et al (2013) Ovarian response to controlled ovarian hyperstimulation in cancer patients is diminished even before oncological treatment. Fertil Steril 97:930–934. doi:10.1016/j.fertnstert.2012.01.093

70. Cakmak H, Katz A, Cedars MI et al (2013) Effective method for emergency fertility preservation: random-start controlled ovarian stimulation. Fertil Steril 100:1673–1680. doi:10.1016/j.fertnstert.2013.07.1992
71. Kuang Y, Hong Q, Chen Q et al (2014) Luteal-phase ovarian stimulation is feasible for producing competent oocytes in women undergoing in vitro fertilization/intracytoplasmic sperm injection treatment, with optimal pregnancy outcomes in frozen-thawed embryo transfer cycles. Fertil Steril 101:105–111. doi:10.1016/j.fertnstert.2013.09.007
72. García-Velasco JA, Domingo J, Cobo A et al (2013) 5-years experience employing oocyte vitrification to preserve fertility for medical and non-medical indications. Fertil Steril 99:1994–1999. doi:10.1016/j.fertnstert.2013.02.004
73. Cil AP, Bang H, Oktay K (2013) Age-specific probability of live birth with oocyte cryopreservation: an individual patient data meta-analysis. Fertil Steril 100:492–499. doi:10.1016/j.fertnstert.2013.04.023
74. Lawrenz B, Jauckus J, Kupka MS et al (2011) Fertility preservation in >1,000 patients: patient's characteristics, spectrum, efficacy and risks of applied preservation techniques. Arch Gynecol Obstet 283:651–656. doi:10.1007/s00404-010-1772-y

Chapter 2
Controlled Ovarian Stimulation Protocols in Cancer Patients

Hakan Cakmak and Mitchell P. Rosen

Abstract Embryo/oocyte cryopreservation is an effective method for fertility preservation in cancer patients. Determination of the controlled ovarian stimulation protocol and gonadotropin dose for oocyte/embryo cryopreservation requires an individualized assessment. Maximizing the number of embryos and oocytes cryopreserved during a fertility preservation cycle without causing ovarian hyperstimulation syndrome is extremely important, because the most of the patients have a single cycle opportunity due to time constraints before starting their oncologic treatment. In emergent settings, random-start ovarian stimulation is emerging as a new technique for the purpose of fertility preservation without compromising oocyte yield and maturity. Ovarian stimulation with tamoxifen or letrozole is highly recommended in patients with estrogen-sensitive cancers undergoing fertility preservation. While only a minority of the cancer patients has undergone thawing and embryo transfer, recent data of these modified protocols in egg donors and infertile patients have suggested that pregnancy outcomes are similar to those of conventional protocols.

Keywords Cancer • Controlled ovarian stimulation • Random-start ovarian stimulation • Fertility preservation • Oocyte/embryo cryopreservation

2.1 Introduction

Cancer is no longer considered as incurable disease among reproductive age women. Over the past decades, there has been a remarkable improvement in the survival rates due to the marked progress in detecting cancer at earlier stages and the improvement in treatment modalities [1]. Between 2002 and 2012, 83 % of women younger than 45 years diagnosed with cancer survived [1]. As a consequence of the increase in the number of cancer survivors, quality of life issues such

H. Cakmak (✉) • M.P. Rosen
Division of Reproductive Endocrinology and Infertility, Department of Obstetrics, Gynecology, and Reproductive Sciences, University of California San Francisco, 6th Floor, 499 Illinois Street, San Francisco, CA 94158, USA
e-mail: hakan.cakmak@ucsf.edu

N. Suzuki, J. Donnez (eds.), *Gonadal Tissue Cryopreservation in Fertility Preservation*, DOI 10.1007/978-4-431-55963-4_2

as fertility preservation have become paramount in the lives of reproductive age women battling malignancy and an integral component in cancer management [2, 3].

The treatment for most of the cancer types in reproductive age women involves either removal of the reproductive organs or cytotoxic treatment (chemotherapy and/or radiotherapy) [4]. The irreversible gonadotoxic effects of some of the chemotherapeutic agents are well documented, particularly for alkylating agents, which are common components of chemotherapy for breast cancer, lymphomas, leukemia, and sarcomas [5, 6]. Pelvic radiation therapy also causes follicular destruction, and less than 2 Gy of radiation can deplete at least 50 % of the follicles [7]. In addition, exposure to 5–10 Gy of pelvic radiation results in premature ovarian insufficiency in many women [4]. The risk of ovarian failure following cancer therapy appears to be dose related, and the effect is dependent on age and ovarian reserve at the time of treatment [8].

Early loss of ovarian function not only puts the patients at risk for menopause-related complications at a very young age but is also associated with loss of fertility [5]. Multiple strategies have emerged aiming to preserve fertility in females with different types of malignancies. Controlled ovarian stimulation (COS) for embryo or mature oocyte cryopreservation is an effective method for fertility preservation in cancer patients due to its potential for high success rates compared to other more experimental technologies and is the only technique endorsed by the American Society of Reproductive Medicine (ASRM) [9, 10]. Therefore, it should be recommended as long as the patient's medical condition does not preclude safely performing COS or oocyte retrieval; and the patient has adequate time to undergo COS and oocyte retrieval [9, 10].

2.2 Conventional COS Protocols

Conventionally, ovarian stimulation for oocyte/embryo cryopreservation is initiated at the beginning of the follicular phase with the idea that this optimizes clinical outcomes. The treatment time for ovarian stimulation ranges from 9 to 14 days with either a GnRH agonist or antagonists to suppress ovulation. Although multiple different COS protocols are being used, the majority of cancer patients are treated with a GnRH antagonist-based protocol (Fig. 2.1a), which likely allows the shortest deferral of the initiation of cancer treatment [11]. This may be due to less ovarian suppression with use of GnRH antagonists compared to agonists [12]. Another reason is that, compared to GnRH agonists, GnRH antagonists are rapid acting to suppress pituitary release of gonadotropins. Typically, GnRH antagonists are initiated to prevent premature LH surge when the lead follicle reaches to 12–14 mm at approximately day 6 of gonadotropin stimulation. In contrast, GnRH agonist may require a pretreatment phase to downregulate GnRH receptors prior to the administration of gonadotropins which adds to the total treatment time.

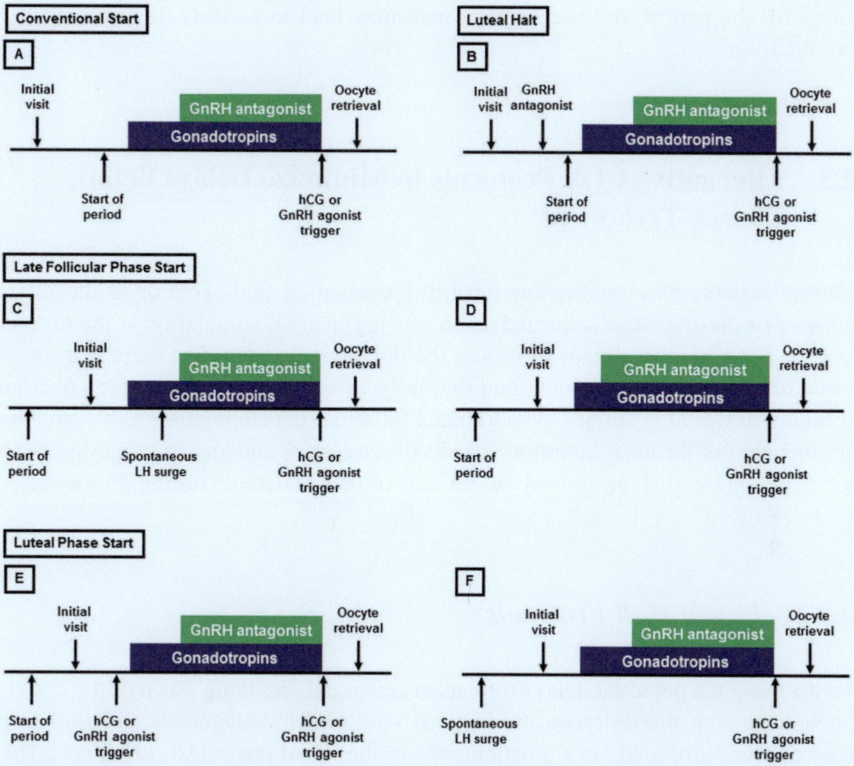

Fig. 2.1 Controlled ovarian stimulation protocols in cancer patients. (**a**) In conventional (early follicular phase start) antagonist protocol, ovarian stimulation starts with menses, and GnRH antagonist is initiated when the lead follicle reaches 12 mm. (**b**) In luteal halt protocol, administration of GnRH antagonist in the luteal phase induces corpus luteum regression, menses ensues 2–4 days later, and ovarian stimulation is initiated earlier than awaiting spontaneous menses. If the cancer patient presents in the late follicular phase, (**c**) ovarian stimulation without GnRH antagonist can be started if the follicle cohort following the lead follicle is smaller than 12 mm and stays smaller than 12 mm before a spontaneous LH surge. After the LH surge, GnRH antagonist is started when the secondary follicle cohort reaches 12 mm to prevent premature secondary LH surge. (**d**) If the follicle cohort following the lead follicle reaches 12 mm *before* the spontaneous LH surge, pituitary suppression with GnRH antagonist is initiated and continued until triggering final oocyte maturation. If the cancer patient presents in the late follicular phase, (**e**) ovulation can be induced with hCG or GnRH agonist when the dominant follicle reaches to 18 mm in diameter and ovarian stimulation is started in 2–3 days in luteal phase. If the cancer patient presents in the luteal phase, (**f**) ovarian stimulation can be started in the absence of GnRH antagonist, and GnRH antagonist administration is initiated later in the cycle, when the follicle cohort reached 12 mm to prevent premature secondary LH surge

This methodology may require 2–6 weeks depending on the women's menstrual cycle phase at the time of presentation. As a result, there remains the possibility of a significant delay of cancer treatment and the potential for increased psychological stress for the patient and oncologist which may lead to patients forgoing fertility preservation.

2.3 Alternative COS Protocols to Minimize Delays Before Cancer Treatment

Cancer patients may present for fertility preservation mid-cycle or in the luteal phase. For these patients, alternatives to starting ovarian stimulation at the time of menses have been explored. However, the dogma suggesting that there is a single wave of follicular development and that only early follicular phase starts ovarian stimulation would result in a synchronized follicular development [13, 14], and the strong belief of the local inhibitory effects of the corpus luteum and progesterone in the luteal phase [15] questioned the success of these alternate timing protocols.

2.3.1 Luteal Halt Protocols

To decrease the potential delays for cancer treatment, breaking down of the corpus luteum (to stop progesterone production) with GnRH antagonists and initiating menses were proposed once a patient was in the luteal phase [16, 17] (Fig. 2.1b). The studies showed that after the administration of GnRH antagonist in the luteal phase (e.g., a single 3 mg dose or two to three consecutive daily 250 μg doses), serum progesterone levels decreased and menses ensued 2–4 days later [16, 17]. As a result, ovarian stimulation would be initiated earlier than awaiting spontaneous menses. GnRH antagonist would be restarted in a standard fashion to prevent premature LH surge during ovarian stimulation [17]. Although there are few studies, the evidence suggests a synchronized follicle development and expected mature oocyte yield with normal fertilization rates and embryo quality.

In another protocol, GnRH antagonists and recombinant FSH were administered simultaneously during the luteal phase of the menstrual cycle and have observed shorter treatment times due to not awaiting for menses [18]. Only FSH was used for follicular stimulation to avoid exogenous LH activity which might prevent luteolysis. Compared to the cancer patients stimulated throughout the follicular phase ($n = 28$), the luteal-phase group ($n = 12$) had a similar number of mature oocytes as well as comparable fertilization rates [18]. In the same study, it was also shown that in several patients whose ovarian stimulation started in late follicular phase, the oocyte recovery and normal fertilization were possible.

2.3.2 Random-Start (Late Follicular or Luteal-Phase Start) COS Protocols

Another alternative approach is to initiate ovarian stimulation regardless of the menstrual phase (i.e., random-start COS) [19–25].

Initial case reports and series on random-start COS have been published with encouraging results [20–22, 24]. A report of three breast cancer patients evaluated the effectiveness of initiating ovarian stimulation at the time of patient presentation (menstrual cycle day 11, 14, and 17) rather than waiting for spontaneous menses [20]. The random-start ovarian stimulation was resulted in a reasonable ovarian response with seven to ten embryos cryopreserved per patient [20]. In another case report, two cancer patients had successful COS initiated during the luteal phase that resulted in retrieval of 12 MII oocytes in both cases [21]. The patient with Hodgkin lymphoma, who underwent random-start COS starting on day 11 of her menstrual cycle with the use of the GnRH antagonist initiating simultaneously with ovarian stimulation, had 17 mature oocytes cryopreserved [24].

The report presenting our clinical experience on random-start ovarian stimulation demonstrated that late follicular or luteal-phase start COS were as effective as early follicular start COS in cancer patients [19].

If the cancer patient presented in the late follicular phase, one of the following treatment plans was performed:

(a) COS *without* GnRH antagonist was started if the follicle cohort following the lead follicle was smaller than 12 mm and stayed smaller than 12 mm before a spontaneous LH surge (Fig. 2.1c). After the LH surge, GnRH antagonist was started when the secondary follicle cohort reached 12 mm to prevent premature secondary LH surge (Fig. 2.1c). If the follicle cohort following the lead follicle reached 12 mm *before* the spontaneous LH surge, pituitary suppression with GnRH antagonist was initiated and continued until triggering final oocyte maturation (Fig. 2.1d)
(b) Ovulation was induced with hCG or GnRH agonist when the dominant follicle reached 18 mm in diameter, and ovarian stimulation was started in 2–3 days in luteal phase (Fig. 2.1d) [19].

If the cancer patient presented in the luteal phase or the ovulation was induced, ovarian stimulation was started in the *absence* of GnRH antagonist (Fig. 2.1e, f). Similar to conventional COS, GnRH antagonist administration was initiated later in the cycle, when the follicle cohort reached 12 mm to prevent premature secondary LH surge.

The number of mature oocytes retrieved (9.7 versus 9.9) and fertilization rates (72 % versus 87 %) were similar in early follicular start and random-start protocols [19]. Moreover, starting COS in the late follicular or luteal phase did not show any superiority against the other [19]. Subsequent studies supported our findings and also demonstrated the efficiency of random-start COS [23, 25].

In contrast to previous belief, the presence of corpus luteum or luteal-phase progesterone levels did not adversely affect synchronized follicular development, number of mature oocytes retrieved, and/or fertilization rates [19, 26]. Because spontaneous corpus luteum regression occurs possibly due to suppressive effect of rising estradiol levels on endogenous LH secretion during COS, corpus luteum regression with GnRH antagonist was not necessary to start COS [19]. The length of the cycle and daily gonadotropin dose were not affected by the serum progesterone level or whether COS was started in the early or mid-luteal phase [19, 26]. In addition, the ovary with corpus luteum had similar number of dominant follicles ($\geq$13 mm) compared to patient's other ovary on the day of trigger shot [26].

Overall, random-start ovarian stimulation provides a significant advantage by decreasing total time for the IVF cycle, and in emergent settings, COS can be started at a random cycle date for the purpose of fertility preservation without compromising oocyte yield and maturity. Although random-start COS protocols are efficient in obtaining appropriate number of mature oocytes/embryos, only a minority of the cancer patients underwent thawing and embryo transfer, and therefore, there is not enough reported data to evaluate the implantation rate and pregnancy rates in cancer patients.

However, comparable pregnancy rates and outcomes after transferring embryos created from infertile patients and egg donors with late follicular and luteal-phase start protocols are encouraging [27–30]. In a study comparing the pregnancy outcomes in recipients of embryos from donor oocytes obtained after COS initiated in early proliferative phase (day 2 of menstrual phase) versus in luteal phase (day 15 of menstrual phase), there were no differences noted in pregnancy (62 % versus 58 %) or implantation rates (41 % versus 45 %) [30]. In a small self-controlled clinical trial, egg donors underwent COS starting in early follicular phase followed by another COS cycle initiated on either day 10 (late follicular phase) or on day 20 (luteal phase) of the menstrual cycle [27]. The alternate timing ovarian stimulation resulted in similar number of mature oocytes, fertilization rate, and number of good quality embryos with appropriate clinical pregnancy rates compared to conventional (early follicular start) protocol [27]. In infertile women undergoing IVF, COS after spontaneous ovulation (i.e., luteal-phase start) followed by embryo cryopreservation and frozen embryo transfer resulted in comparable clinical pregnancy rate (55 %), ongoing pregnancy rate (49 %), and implantation rate (40 %) [29] with similar pregnancy outcomes and no increase in congenital birth defects [28]. Additional clinical studies are needed to further assess the efficacy of this strategy in cancer patients.

2.4 Controlled Ovarian Stimulation in Patients with Estrogen-Sensitive Cancers

During COS, the supraphysiological estrogen levels as a result of ovarian stimulation with gonadotropins may promote the growth of estrogen-sensitive tumors such as endometrial and estrogen receptor-positive breast cancers [31]. The rise in estradiol is directly proportional to the number of growing follicles; therefore, alternative and potentially safer protocols have been introduced for fertility preservation for estrogen-sensitive cancer patients including natural cycle IVF (without ovarian stimulation) and stimulation protocols with tamoxifen/aromatase inhibitors alone or combined with gonadotropins [32].

Natural cycle IVF only gives one or two oocytes or embryos per cycle and has high risk of not having oocytes or embryos to freeze due to premature ovulation, not able to obtain any oocytes during retrieval and fertilization failures. Therefore, this technique would likely be ineffective and is not recommended especially when a gonadotoxic treatment is imminent and the patient does not have a chance for a second cycle of IVF treatment.

Tamoxifen and its metabolites have a well-known antiestrogenic action on breast tissue with the inhibition of growth of breast tumors by competitive antagonism of estrogen at its receptor site and are accepted as the first-line drug in hormonal prevention and treatment of estrogen receptor-positive breast cancer [33]. Tamoxifen, besides its effect in the breast, has also an antagonist action in the estrogen receptors in the central nervous system similar to that of clomiphene. The selective antagonist action of tamoxifen interferes with the negative feedback of the estrogen on the hypothalamic/pituitary axis leading to an increase in GnRH secretion from the hypothalamus and a subsequent release of FSH from the pituitary stimulating follicular development.

Tamoxifen can be used for COS alone starting on day 2–5 of the menstrual cycle in doses of 20–60 mg/day, or in combination with gonadotropins, similar to the use of clomiphene [32]. Even though peak estradiol levels in ovarian stimulation with tamoxifen are not altered, due to its antiestrogenic effect on breast tissue, it is desirable to be used in estrogen-receptor-positive breast cancer patients. Studies using tamoxifen during ovarian stimulation showed no adverse effect of tamoxifen on oocyte and embryo development [34, 35]. Ovarian stimulation using tamoxifen for fertility preservation in cancer patients was shown to increase the mature oocyte and embryo yield when compared with natural cycle IVF (1.6 versus 0.7 and 1.6 versus 0.6, respectively) and reduce cycle cancelations [36]. As expected, combined protocol with tamoxifen and gonadotropins further increased the number of cryopreserved oocytes and embryos (5.1 versus 1.5 and 3.8 versus 1.3, respectively) [37]. In breast cancer patients, coadministration of tamoxifen during conventional COS for fertility preservation did not affect the number of oocytes retrieved and embryos stored [35].

Aromatase is a cytochrome P450 enzyme complex that catalyzes the conversion of androstenedione and testosterone to their respective estrogenic products estrone and estradiol [38]. Aromatase inhibitors, such as letrozole, can markedly suppress plasma estrogen levels by competitively inhibiting the activity of the aromatase enzyme [39]. Centrally, aromatase inhibitors release the hypothalamic/pituitary axis from estrogenic negative feedback, increase the secretion of FSH by the pituitary gland, stimulate follicle growth, and, thereby, can be used for ovulation induction [40].

In patients with estrogen-sensitive cancers, the main advantage of adding daily letrozole to gonadotropins in ovarian stimulation protocols is to decrease serum estradiol levels closer to that observed in natural cycles (i.e., estradiol <500 pg/ml) [41, 42]. In a study comparing the efficacy of the letrozole plus gonadotropin protocol in breast cancer patients and the standard IVF protocol in age-matched noncancer patients with tubal factor infertility, the breast cancer patients started to receive letrozole (5 mg/day) on menstrual cycle day 2 or 3, FSH (150–300 IU/day) was added 2 days later, all medications were discontinued on the day of hCG trigger, and letrozole was reinitiated after oocyte retrieval and continued until estradiol levels fell below 50 pg/mL [42]. As expected, peak estradiol levels were significantly lower in the breast cancer patients receiving letrozole plus gonadotropin compared with the standard IVF group (483 ± 279 pg/ml vs. 1,464 ± 645 pg/ml) [42]. This letrozole plus gonadotropin protocol resulted in similar number of total mature oocytes retrieved and length of ovarian stimulation compared to standard IVF protocol [42]. However, the subsequent studies assessing the effect of letrozole on oocyte maturity and competence are controversial, but the data are limited. While some studies demonstrated that the addition of letrozole to the COS protocol improved or did not change the number of mature oocytes retrieved and fertilization rates [43, 44], others showed decrease in mature oocyte yield [45, 46]. Data suggests that the mature oocyte/embryo yield after COS with letrozole is the highest when the lead follicle reaches to 20 mm in diameter (compared to 18 mm in non-letrozole cycles) [42]. In our clinical experience, we do not see any compromise with the use of letrozole in conventional or random-start protocols, if the final oocyte maturation is triggered when the lead follicle reaches to 20 mm in diameter [19, 23].

Letrozole suppresses plasma estradiol levels significantly at doses of 0.1–10 mg/day [47]. In our clinical practice, we start letrozole 2.5 or 5 mg/day, depending on the ovarian reserve of the patient, with the ovarian stimulation. We check estradiol levels in every clinic visit and titrate letrozole dose up to 10 mg/day to keep estradiol levels lower than 500 pg/ml. We also consider continuing letrozole after the oocyte retrieval if serum estradiol levels are still elevated (i.e., estradiol higher than 500 pg/ml). In our experience, even if estradiol levels are above 500 pg/ml prior to retrieval, only a minority of patients requires letrozole post-retrieval. Discontinuation of letrozole can either be at menses or with initiation of chemotherapy. In contrast, anastrozole – another third-generation aromatase inhibitor – failed to adequately suppress estradiol levels during COS despite gradually increasing the dose of anastrozole to a maximum of 10 mg daily, and therefore, we do not recommend its use in fertility preservation cycles [48].

Few studies have evaluated the impact of COS on survival and recurrence of cancer rates in patients with estrogen-sensitive tumors. To date the data has suggested no difference in disease-free survival in patients with breast cancer undergoing ovarian stimulation with the addition of tamoxifen/letrozole even after multiple cycles [35, 37, 49, 50]. In addition, COS with aromatase inhibitors in combination with gonadotropins was also used with no apparent increased risk for embryo cryopreservation in endometrial cancer patients [51]. However, the studies present certain limitations in methodology, such as the insufficient size of the sample group and the short duration of the monitoring. Therefore, larger studies with longer follow-up are required to evaluate the ongoing safety of COS protocols with tamoxifen/letrozole.

In the early years of the introduction of letrozole as ovarian stimulants, concerns were raised on the potential impact of the treatment on the resulting pregnancy, especially given the fact that in an animal study, letrozole was shown to be teratogenic when fetuses were exposed during organogenesis [52]. However, clinical studies did not associate letrozole with birth defects when it was used as an ovulation induction agent. The study assessing 911 babies born after ovulation induction with letrozole or clomiphene for 5 days (from days 3 to 7 of the menstrual cycle) found no differences in the overall rates of fetal malformations or chromosomal abnormalities among newborns of mothers who conceived after letrozole ($n = 514$) or clomiphene ($n = 397$) treatments [53]. In another study, in which 750 women with polycystic ovary syndrome were randomly assigned to receive letrozole or clomiphene for ovulation induction, similar rates of major congenital anomalies in the letrozole (4 of 102) and clomiphene group (1 of 66) were reported [54].

In a recent study, it was demonstrated that the pregnancy outcomes of frozen embryo transfers with embryos generated after ovarian stimulation with letrozole in patients with breast cancer were comparable (65 % clinical pregnancy rate (26 of 40) with 45 % live birth rate (18 of 40)) to those of infertile women in the same age category [55]. A total of 25 babies were born from 18 pregnancies of which 38.8 % (7 of 18) were twins. The mean gestational age was 38.0 ± 2.3 weeks. Additionally, after a mean follow-up of more than 3 years, no minor or major fetal malformations or developmental abnormalities were observed in the newborn [55]. These are not surprising findings given that letrozole has a short (48 h) half-life and the cryopreserved embryos generated in vitro have no direct exposure to letrozole. Currently, no data is available about the pregnancy outcomes of frozen embryo transfers with embryos generated after COS with tamoxifen in cancer patients.

In summary, COS with tamoxifen and/or letrozole plus gonadotropins in patients with estrogen-sensitive cancers undergoing fertility preservation is equally well tolerated and yields similar number of oocytes and embryos compared to standard protocols while minimizing the risk of high estrogen exposure. Although there are no data to suggest that ovarian stimulation without these estrogen modulators leads to progression of disease, there is biologic plausibility of increased risk. Therefore, we highly recommend the routine use of tamoxifen and/or letrozole during COS for fertility preservation in patients with estrogen-sensitive cancers.

2.5 Response to Ovarian Stimulation in Cancer Patients

In cancer patients, both the specific malignancy and the patient's multisystemic condition may have an impact on the response to ovarian stimulation [56]. The increased catabolic state, malnutrition, and increased stress hormone levels associated with the malignancy may affect the hypothalamic-gonadal axis and negatively impact ovarian reserve or oocyte quality [57–59]. There are mixed reports about how cancer patients respond to COS protocols; while some are reporting no significant change [60–62], others demonstrate worse ovarian response in cancer patients compared to age-matched healthy women [59, 63]. In a meta-analysis of seven retrospective studies, women with malignancies had lower number of total oocytes (11.7 ± 7.5 vs. 13.5 ± 8.4) and mature oocytes retrieved (9.0 ± 6.5 vs. 10.8 ± 6.8) after COS compared with healthy, age-matched patients [56].

It is well established that AFC correlates directly with number of follicles, number of mature oocytes retrieved, and number of embryos obtained during an IVF cycle [64]. In our clinical experience, although the number of mature oocytes retrieved and embryos may be lower in cancer patients compared to healthy individuals, they are appropriate for their given AFC. Moreover, their response to the gonadotropins and mature oocyte yield (i.e., number of metaphase II oocytes/AFC) is similar to the healthy women. Therefore, if lower oocyte and embryo numbers in patients with malignancy during an IVF cycle are true, this is not due to poor response to ovarian stimulation, but is likely the result of decreased number of available antral follicles to be stimulated.

2.6 Prevention of Ovarian Hyperstimulation Syndrome (OHSS) in Cancer Patients

Ovarian hyperstimulation syndrome (OHSS) is the most serious complication of COS and can be associated with ascites, intravascular depletion, electrolyte imbalance, pulmonary edema, liver dysfunction, and thromboembolic events. Although it is often self-limited with spontaneous resolution within a few days, severe OHSS may require hospitalization and intensive care. The impact of OHSS can be profound in cancer patients, because it may result in delaying or complicating planned lifesaving cancer therapy [65].

Selecting the appropriate ovarian stimulation regimen can be challenging in embryo/oocyte cryopreservation because it is important to balance the risk of OHSS and obtain sufficient number of oocytes or embryos to maximize the chance of a successful pregnancy in the future. Triggering the final oocyte maturation with human chorionic gonadotropin (hCG) carries the well-known risk of inducing OHSS [66]. Using a lower dose of hCG (as low as 3300 IU) can be a strategy to decrease the risk of OHSS without negatively impacting the mature oocyte yield. As an alternative approach, GnRH agonist can be used to induce the final oocyte maturation by promoting the release of endogenous gonadotropins from the hypophysis as long as the pituitary GnRH receptors are not downregulated [66]. GnRH agonist trigger in GnRH-antagonist-based protocols dramatically reduces the risk of OHSS due to the short half-life of GnRH agonist-induced endogenous LH surge [67]. In addition, significantly lower rate of moderate/severe OHSS in the GnRH agonist group was observed compared with the patients who received hCG trigger (2–3 % versus 14–21 %) [68, 69]. GnRH agonist trigger is particularly convenient in cancer patients pursuing oocyte or embryo banking because luteal support is not needed to sustain a pregnancy and GnRH agonist trigger results in at least similar number of mature oocytes and cryopreserved embryos compared with the hCG group [68, 69].

In our experience, trigger failures with GnRH agonist (especially with 1 mg leuprolide acetate dosing) may occur. The likely etiology is that GnRH agonist is able to bind to only a portion of the receptors due to competition with GnRH antagonist yielding a limited LH surge [70]. Increasing the dose of GnRH agonist (up to 4 mg of leuprolide acetate) or adding hCG supplementation (1,500 IU) at the time of trigger may result in less failures. Due to the possibility of failure, we do not routinely administer GnRH agonist trigger for all patients. In our current practice, 4 mg of leuprolide acetate is being used only in patients with high risk of OHSS. If the patient has known hypothalamic dysfunction and has high risk of OHSS, in our limited clinical experience, very low dose hCG (1,500 IU) trigger with FSH supplementation (450 IU) at the time of trigger can be an alternative without negatively impacting the mature oocyte yield.

The number of follicles in combination with serum estradiol levels predicts OHSS with high sensitivity and specificity [71, 72]. However, co-treatment with aromatase inhibitors limits the utilization of serum estradiol level to predict OHSS. In this scenario, it is important to rely on the follicular pattern and the rate of estradiol rise rather than the absolute serum estradiol levels. If the estradiol levels are rising rapidly while administering letrozole especially in the presence of a high number of small follicles, the patient should be considered as being at risk of OHSS, and GnRH agonist trigger should be used to lower this risk.

In conclusion, we recommend GnRH agonist trigger in GnRH antagonist-based cycles only for women who are at risk for OHSS. The success of trigger must be confirmed the next morning by measuring serum LH level. In the case of a GnRH agonist trigger failure determined by low post-trigger LH (in our clinic, we use the cut-off LH level less than 12 mIU/ml), hCG (3,300–5,000 IU) trigger can be given on the same day [73]. If the patient has relatively low post-trigger LH level, but higher than 12 mIU/ml, the closer attention should be given to the oocyte yield during the oocyte retrieval. If no or inappropriately low number of oocytes are retrieved after aspirating a couple of mature size follicles, the oocyte retrieval should be stopped, oocyte maturation should be triggered again by administering hCG (3,300–5,000 IU) due to the possibility of failing to trigger oocyte maturation with GnRH agonist, and then oocyte retrieval should be attempted again 36 h later [73].

2.7 Timing of Ovarian Stimulation

In order to perform a successful oocyte/embryo cryopreservation cycle, the treating fertility specialist must remain cognizant of time constraints surrounding the patient's cancer treatment. In patients with hematological malignancies (i.e., leukemia and lymphoma), the tumor burden is generally high at the outset of diagnosis, requiring that cancer therapy begins almost immediately. Therefore, in these patients, random-start COS can be initiated immediately after the initial visit start, and delays to the cancer treatment can be minimized.

In other cancer types where the surgery is the first step in tumor management (e.g., breast cancer), the patient may have 4–6-week window before or between surgery and adjuvant therapy. In these cases, ovarian stimulation and oocyte/embryo cryopreservation can be performed before and/or immediately after the surgery, and thereafter patients can proceed with surgery or additional cancer treatment (i.e., chemo, radiation, and/or hormonal therapy).

In patients with low ovarian reserve, predispositions to genetic conditions, and patients of older age, it may be beneficial to do multiple cycles prior to cancer treatment to obtain more oocytes/embryos to improve the chance of pregnancy. The timing of these multiple ovarian stimulations can either be based on cancer treatment windows (i.e., prior to or after surgery and prior to chemotherapy) or possibly be done one after the other. Studies indicate that there are more than one follicle recruitment wave during a menstrual cycle [74]. Therefore, to minimize delays, an ovarian stimulation can be started a couple of days after egg retrieval (i.e., in luteal phase). With this approach, mature eggs and cleavage stage embryos were obtained in poor responders [75, 76]. Although effective with patients with poor ovarian reserve, there is limited data on the effectiveness with patients that have good ovarian reserve and/or with persistent cysts left over from the prior stimulation.

2.8 Conclusions

Embryo cryopreservation is an effective method for fertility preservation, and oocyte cryopreservation has gained efficacy and is now offered at many centers. Determination of the COS protocol and gonadotropin dose for oocyte/embryo cryopreservation requires an individualized assessment. Maximizing the number of embryos and oocytes cryopreserved during a fertility preservation cycle without causing OHSS is extremely important, because most of the patients have a single cycle opportunity due to time constraints before starting their oncologic treatment. In emergent settings, random-start ovarian stimulation is emerging as a new technique for the purpose of fertility preservation without compromising oocyte yield and maturity. COS with tamoxifen or letrozole is highly recommended in patients with estrogen-sensitive cancers undergoing fertility preservation. While only a minority of the cancer patients have undergone thawing and embryo transfer, recent data of these modified protocols in the infertile patient has suggested that pregnancy outcomes are similar to those of conventional protocols. More studies are needed to confirm these findings. However, with the available data, we should be reassured that random-start protocols with or without estrogen modulation is an effective treatment for fertility preservation and should minimize anxieties about delaying cancer treatment and enable most patients with cancer an opportunity to preserve their reproductive potential.

References

1. Howlader N, Noone AM, Krapcho M, Neyman N, Aminou R, Waldron W, Altekruse SF, Kosary CL, Ruhl J, Tatalovich Z, Cho H, Mariotto A, Eisner MP, Lewis DR, Chen HS, Feuer EJ, Cronin KA (eds). SEER cancer statistics review, 1975–2009 (Vintage 2009 populations), National Cancer Institute. Bethesda. Available at: http://seer.cancer.gov/csr/1975_2009_pops09/. Accessed on 16 June 2015
2. Letourneau JM, Ebbel EE, Katz PP, Katz A, Ai WZ, Chien AJ, Melisko ME, Cedars MI, Rosen MP (2012) Pretreatment fertility counseling and fertility preservation improve quality of life in reproductive age women with cancer. Cancer 118(6):1710–1717
3. Letourneau JM, Melisko ME, Cedars MI, Rosen MP (2011) A changing perspective: improving access to fertility preservation. Nat Rev Clin Oncol 8(1):56–60
4. Rodriguez-Wallberg KA, Oktay K (2012) Options on fertility preservation in female cancer patients. Cancer Treat Rev 38(5):354–361
5. Letourneau JM, Ebbel EE, Katz PP, Oktay KH, McCulloch CE, Ai WZ, Chien AJ, Melisko ME, Cedars MI, Rosen MP (2012) Acute ovarian failure underestimates age-specific reproductive impairment for young women undergoing chemotherapy for cancer. Cancer 118 (7):1933–1939
6. Maltaris T, Seufert R, Fischl F, Schaffrath M, Pollow K, Koelbl H, Dittrich R (2007) The effect of cancer treatment on female fertility and strategies for preserving fertility. Eur J Obstet Gynecol Reprod Biol 130(2):148–155
7. Wallace WH, Thomson AB, Kelsey TW (2003) The radiosensitivity of the human oocyte. Hum Reprod 18(1):117–121
8. Meirow D, Nugent D (2001) The effects of radiotherapy and chemotherapy on female reproduction. Hum Reprod Update 7(6):535–543
9. The Practice Committee of the American Society for Reproductive Medicine (2005) Fertility preservation and reproduction in cancer patients. Fertil Steril 83(6):1622–1628
10. The Practice Committee of the American Society for Reproductive Medicine (2013) Mature oocyte cryopreservation: a guideline. Fertil Steril 99(1):37–43
11. McLaren JF, Bates GW (2012) Fertility preservation in women of reproductive age with cancer. Am J Obstet Gynecol 207(6):455–462
12. Schachter M, Friedler S, Raziel A, Strassburger D, Bern O, Ron-el R (2001) Improvement of IVF outcome in poor responders by discontinuation of GnRH analogue during the gonadotropin stimulation phase – a function of improved embryo quality. J Assist Reprod Genet 18 (4):197–204
13. Gougeon A (1986) Dynamics of follicular growth in the human: a model from preliminary results. Hum Reprod 1(2):81–87
14. Pache TD, Wladimiroff JW, de Jong FH, Hop WC, Fauser BC (1990) Growth patterns of nondominant ovarian follicles during the normal menstrual cycle. Fertil Steril 54(4):638–642

15. McNatty KP, Hillier SG, van den Boogaard AM, Trimbos-Kemper TC, Reichert LE Jr, van Hall EV (1983) Follicular development during the luteal phase of the human menstrual cycle. J Clin Endocrinol Metab 56(5):1022–1031
16. Anderson RA, Kinniburgh D, Baird DT (1999) Preliminary experience of the use of a gonadotropin-releasing hormone antagonist in ovulation induction/in-vitro fertilization prior to cancer treatment. Hum Reprod 14(10):2665–2668
17. Humaidan P, Bungum L, Bungum M, Hald F, Agerholm I, Blaabjerg J, Yding Andersen C, Lindenberg S (2005) Reproductive outcome using a GnRH antagonist (cetrorelix) for luteolysis and follicular synchronization in poor responder IVF/ICSI patients treated with a flexible GnRH antagonist protocol. Reprod Biomed Online 11(6):679–684
18. von Wolff M, Thaler CJ, Frambach T, Zeeb C, Lawrenz B, Popovici RM, Strowitzki T (2009) Ovarian stimulation to cryopreserve fertilized oocytes in cancer patients can be started in the luteal phase. Fertil Steril 92(4):1360–1365
19. Cakmak H, Katz A, Cedars MI, Rosen MP (2013) Effective method for emergency fertility preservation: random-start controlled ovarian stimulation. Fertil Steril 100(6):1673–1680. doi:10.1016/j.fertnstert.2013.07.1992
20. Sonmezer M, Turkcuoglu I, Coskun U, Oktay K (2011) Random-start controlled ovarian hyperstimulation for emergency fertility preservation in letrozole cycles. Fertil Steril 95 (6):2125, e2129–2111
21. Bedoschi GM, de Albuquerque FO, Ferriani RA, Navarro PA (2010) Ovarian stimulation during the luteal phase for fertility preservation of cancer patients: case reports and review of the literature. J Assist Reprod Genet 27(8):491–494
22. Nayak SR, Wakim AN (2011) Random-start gonadotropin-releasing hormone (GnRH) antagonist-treated cycles with GnRH agonist trigger for fertility preservation. Fertil Steril 96 (1):e51–e54. doi:10.1016/j.fertnstert.2011.04.079
23. Keskin U, Ercan CM, Yilmaz A, Babacan A, Korkmaz C, Duru NK, Ergun A (2014) Random-start controlled ovarian hyperstimulation with letrozole for fertility preservation in cancer patients: case series and review of literature. J Pak Med Assoc 64(7):830–832
24. Ozkaya E, San Roman G, Oktay K (2012) Luteal phase GnRHa trigger in random start fertility preservation cycles. J Assist Reprod Genet 29(6):503–505. doi:10.1007/s10815-012-9752-8
25. Kim JH, Kim SK, Lee HJ, Lee JR, Jee BC, Suh CS, Kim SH (2015) Efficacy of random-start controlled ovarian stimulation in cancer patients. J Korean Med Sci 30(3):290–295. doi:10.3346/jkms.2015.30.3.290
26. Cakmak H, Mok-Lin E, Katz A, Harris E, Chin-Yu C, Cedars MI, Rosen MP (2014) Random start controlled ovarian stimulation results in high oocyte developmental competence and embryo quality. Fertil Steril 102(3):e164
27. Checa MA, Brassesco M, Sastre M, Gomez M, Herrero J, Marque L, Brassesco A, Espinos JJ (2015) Random-start GnRH antagonist for emergency fertility preservation: a self-controlled trial. Int J Womens Health 7:219–225. doi:10.2147/IJWH.S66743
28. Chen H, Wang Y, Lyu Q, Ai A, Fu Y, Tian H, Cai R, Hong Q, Chen Q, Shoham Z, Kuang Y (2015) Comparison of live-birth defects after luteal-phase ovarian stimulation vs. conventional ovarian stimulation for in vitro fertilization and vitrified embryo transfer cycles. Fertil Steril 103(5):1194–1201 e1192. doi:10.1016/j.fertnstert.2015.02.020
29. Kuang Y, Hong Q, Chen Q, Lyu Q, Ai A, Fu Y, Shoham Z (2014) Luteal-phase ovarian stimulation is feasible for producing competent oocytes in women undergoing in vitro fertilization/intracytoplasmic sperm injection treatment, with optimal pregnancy outcomes in frozen-thawed embryo transfer cycles. Fertil Steril 101(1):105–111. doi:10.1016/j.fertnstert.2013.09.007
30. Martinez F, Clua E, Devesa M, Rodriguez I, Arroyo G, Gonzalez C, Sole M, Tur R, Coroleu B, Barri PN (2014) Comparison of starting ovarian stimulation on day 2 versus day 15 of the menstrual cycle in the same oocyte donor and pregnancy rates among the corresponding recipients of vitrified oocytes. Fertil Steril 102(5):1307–1311. doi:10.1016/j.fertnstert.2014.07.741

31. Reddy J, Oktay K (2012) Ovarian stimulation and fertility preservation with the use of aromatase inhibitors in women with breast cancer. Fertil Steril 98(6):1363–1369
32. Rodriguez-Wallberg KA, Oktay K (2010) Fertility preservation in women with breast cancer. Clin Obstet Gynecol 53(4):753–762
33. (1992) Systemic treatment of early breast cancer by hormonal, cytotoxic, or immune therapy. 133 randomised trials involving 31,000 recurrences and 24,000 deaths among 75,000 women. Early Breast Cancer Trialists' Collaborative Group. Lancet 339(8785):71–85
34. Fisk NM, Templeton AA, Papadopoulos GC, Matlin SA, Wu ZY (1989) Lack of effect of high-dose antioestrogen on the maturation and in-vitro fertilization of human oocytes. Hum Reprod 4(5):584–587
35. Meirow D, Raanani H, Maman E, Paluch-Shimon S, Shapira M, Cohen Y, Kuchuk I, Hourvitz A, Levron J, Mozer-Mendel M, Brengauz M, Biderman H, Manela D, Catane R, Dor J, Orvieto R, Kaufman B (2014) Tamoxifen co-administration during controlled ovarian hyperstimulation for in vitro fertilization in breast cancer patients increases the safety of fertility-preservation treatment strategies. Fertil Steril 102(2):488–495 e483. doi:10.1016/j.fertnstert.2014.05.017
36. Oktay K, Buyuk E, Davis O, Yermakova I, Veeck L, Rosenwaks Z (2003) Fertility preservation in breast cancer patients: IVF and embryo cryopreservation after ovarian stimulation with tamoxifen. Hum Reprod 18(1):90–95
37. Oktay K, Buyuk E, Libertella N, Akar M, Rosenwaks Z (2005) Fertility preservation in breast cancer patients: a prospective controlled comparison of ovarian stimulation with tamoxifen and letrozole for embryo cryopreservation. J Clin Oncol 23(19):4347–4353
38. Cole PA, Robinson CH (1990) Mechanism and inhibition of cytochrome P-450 aromatase. J Med Chem 33(11):2933–2942
39. Smith IE, Dowsett M (2003) Aromatase inhibitors in breast cancer. N Engl J Med 348 (24):2431–2442
40. Mitwally MF, Casper RF (2001) Use of an aromatase inhibitor for induction of ovulation in patients with an inadequate response to clomiphene citrate. Fertil Steril 75(2):305–309
41. Testart J, Frydman R, Nahoul K, Grenier J, Feinstein MC, Roger M, Scholler R (1982) Steroids and gonadotropins during the last pre-ovulatory phase of the menstrual cycle. Time relationships between plasma hormones levels and luteinizing hormone surge onset. J Steroid Biochem 17(6):675–682
42. Oktay K, Hourvitz A, Sahin G, Oktem O, Safro B, Cil A, Bang H (2006) Letrozole reduces estrogen and gonadotropin exposure in women with breast cancer undergoing ovarian stimulation before chemotherapy. J Clin Endocrinol Metab 91(10):3885–3890
43. Johnson LN, Dillon KE, Sammel MD, Efymow BL, Mainigi MA, Dokras A, Gracia CR (2013) Response to ovarian stimulation in patients facing gonadotoxic therapy. Reprod Biomed Online 26(4):337–344. doi:10.1016/j.rbmo.2013.01.003
44. Checa Vizcaino MA, Corchado AR, Cuadri ME, Comadran MG, Brassesco M, Carreras R (2012) The effects of letrozole on ovarian stimulation for fertility preservation in cancer-affected women. Reprod Biomed Online 24(6):606–610. doi:10.1016/j.rbmo.2012.02.020
45. Domingo J, Guillen V, Ayllon Y, Martinez M, Munoz E, Pellicer A, Garcia-Velasco JA (2012) Ovarian response to controlled ovarian hyperstimulation in cancer patients is diminished even before oncological treatment. Fertil Steril 97(4):930–934. doi:10.1016/j.fertnstert.2012.01.093
46. Revelli A, Porcu E, Levi Setti PE, Delle Piane L, Merlo DF, Anserini P (2013) Is letrozole needed for controlled ovarian stimulation in patients with estrogen receptor-positive breast cancer? Gynecol Endocrinol 29(11):993–996. doi:10.3109/09513590.2013.819083
47. Klein KO, Demers LM, Santner SJ, Baron J, Cutler GB Jr, Santen RJ (1995) Use of ultrasensitive recombinant cell bioassay to measure estrogen levels in women with breast cancer receiving the aromatase inhibitor, letrozole. J Clin Endocrinol Metab 80(9):2658–2660
48. Azim AA, Costantini-Ferrando M, Lostritto K, Oktay K (2007) Relative potencies of anastrozole and letrozole to suppress estradiol in breast cancer patients undergoing ovarian stimulation before in vitro fertilization. J Clin Endocrinol Metab 92(6):2197–2200

49. Azim AA, Costantini-Ferrando M, Oktay K (2008) Safety of fertility preservation by ovarian stimulation with letrozole and gonadotropins in patients with breast cancer: a prospective controlled study. J Clin Oncol 26(16):2630–2635
50. Turan V, Bedoschi G, Moy F, Oktay K (2013) Safety and feasibility of performing two consecutive ovarian stimulation cycles with the use of letrozole-gonadotropin protocol for fertility preservation in breast cancer patients. Fertil Steril 100(6):1681–1685 e1681. doi:10.1016/j.fertnstert.2013.08.030
51. Azim A, Oktay K (2007) Letrozole for ovulation induction and fertility preservation by embryo cryopreservation in young women with endometrial carcinoma. Fertil Steril 88 (3):657–664
52. Tiboni GM (2004) Aromatase inhibitors and teratogenesis. Fertil Steril 81(4):1158–1159; author reply 1159. doi:10.1016/j.fertnstert.2004.01.006
53. Tulandi T, Martin J, Al-Fadhli R, Kabli N, Forman R, Hitkari J, Librach C, Greenblatt E, Casper RF (2006) Congenital malformations among 911 newborns conceived after infertility treatment with letrozole or clomiphene citrate. Fertil Steril 85(6):1761–1765. doi:10.1016/j.fertnstert.2006.03.014
54. Legro RS, Brzyski RG, Diamond MP, Coutifaris C, Schlaff WD, Casson P, Christman GM, Huang H, Yan Q, Alvero R, Haisenleder DJ, Barnhart KT, Bates GW, Usadi R, Lucidi S, Baker V, Trussell JC, Krawetz SA, Snyder P, Ohl D, Santoro N, Eisenberg E, Zhang H, Network NRM (2014) Letrozole versus clomiphene for infertility in the polycystic ovary syndrome. N Engl J Med 371(2):119–129. doi:10.1056/NEJMoa1313517
55. Oktay K, Turan V, Bedoschi G, Pacheco FS, Moy F (2015) Fertility preservation success subsequent to concurrent aromatase inhibitor treatment and ovarian stimulation in women with breast cancer. J Clin Oncol. doi:10.1200/JCO.2014.59.3723
56. Friedler S, Koc O, Gidoni Y, Raziel A, Ron-El R (2012) Ovarian response to stimulation for fertility preservation in women with malignant disease: a systematic review and meta-analysis. Fertil Steril 97(1):125–133
57. Agarwal A, Said TM (2004) Implications of systemic malignancies on human fertility. Reprod Biomed Online 9(6):673–679
58. Oktay K, Kim JY, Barad D, Babayev SN (2010) Association of BRCA1 mutations with occult primary ovarian insufficiency: a possible explanation for the link between infertility and breast/ovarian cancer risks. J Clin Oncol 28(2):240–244
59. Pal L, Leykin L, Schifren JL, Isaacson KB, Chang YC, Nikruil N, Chen Z, Toth TL (1998) Malignancy may adversely influence the quality and behaviour of oocytes. Hum Reprod 13 (7):1837–1840
60. Das M, Shehata F, Moria A, Holzer H, Son WY, Tulandi T (2011) Ovarian reserve, response to gonadotropins, and oocyte maturity in women with malignancy. Fertil Steril 96(1):122–125
61. Knopman JM, Noyes N, Talebian S, Krey LC, Grifo JA, Licciardi F (2009) Women with cancer undergoing ART for fertility preservation: a cohort study of their response to exogenous gonadotropins. Fertil Steril 91(4 Suppl):1476–1478
62. Robertson AD, Missmer SA, Ginsburg ES (2011) Embryo yield after in vitro fertilization in women undergoing embryo banking for fertility preservation before chemotherapy. Fertil Steril 95(2):588–591
63. Klock SC, Zhang JX, Kazer RR (2010) Fertility preservation for female cancer patients: early clinical experience. Fertil Steril 94(1):149–155
64. Frattarelli JL, Levi AJ, Miller BT, Segars JH (2003) A prospective assessment of the predictive value of basal antral follicles in in vitro fertilization cycles. Fertil Steril 80(2):350–355
65. Delvigne A, Rozenberg S (2002) Epidemiology and prevention of ovarian hyperstimulation syndrome (OHSS): a review. Hum Reprod Update 8(6):559–577
66. Humaidan P, Kol S, Papanikolaou EG (2011) GnRH agonist for triggering of final oocyte maturation: time for a change of practice? Hum Reprod Update 17(4):510–524
67. Engmann L, DiLuigi A, Schmidt D, Nulsen J, Maier D, Benadiva C (2008) The use of gonadotropin-releasing hormone (GnRH) agonist to induce oocyte maturation after

cotreatment with GnRH antagonist in high-risk patients undergoing in vitro fertilization prevents the risk of ovarian hyperstimulation syndrome: a prospective randomized controlled study. Fertil Steril 89(1):84–91
68. Oktay K, Turkcuoglu I, Rodriguez-Wallberg KA (2010) GnRH agonist trigger for women with breast cancer undergoing fertility preservation by aromatase inhibitor/FSH stimulation. Reprod Biomed Online 20(6):783–788
69. Reddy J, Turan V, Bedoschi G, Moy F, Oktay K (2014) Triggering final oocyte maturation with gonadotropin-releasing hormone agonist (GnRHa) versus human chorionic gonadotropin (hCG) in breast cancer patients undergoing fertility preservation: an extended experience. J Assist Reprod Genet 31(7):927–932. doi:10.1007/s10815-014-0248-6
70. McArdle CA, Franklin J, Green L, Hislop JN (2002) Signalling, cycling and desensitisation of gonadotrophin-releasing hormone receptors. J Endocrinol 173(1):1–11
71. Blankstein J, Shalev J, Saadon T, Kukia EE, Rabinovici J, Pariente C, Lunenfeld B, Serr DM, Mashiach S (1987) Ovarian hyperstimulation syndrome: prediction by number and size of preovulatory ovarian follicles. Fertil Steril 47(4):597–602
72. Papanikolaou EG, Pozzobon C, Kolibianakis EM, Camus M, Tournaye H, Fatemi HM, Van Steirteghem A, Devroey P (2006) Incidence and prediction of ovarian hyperstimulation syndrome in women undergoing gonadotropin-releasing hormone antagonist in vitro fertilization cycles. Fertil Steril 85(1):112–120
73. Cakmak H, Fujimoto VY, Zamah AM, Rosen MP, Tran ND, Cedars MI, Rinaudo PF (2012) Metaphase II (MII) oocytes obtained at different time points in the same in vitro fertilization cycle. J Assist Reprod Genet 29(11):1203–1205
74. Baerwald AR, Adams GP, Pierson RA (2012) Ovarian antral folliculogenesis during the human menstrual cycle: a review. Hum Reprod Update 18(1):73–91. doi:10.1093/humupd/dmr039
75. Xu B, Li Y (2013) Flexible ovarian stimulation in a poor responder: a case report and literature review. Reprod Biomed Online 26(4):378–383. doi:10.1016/j.rbmo.2012.11.020
76. Kuang Y, Chen Q, Hong Q, Lyu Q, Ai A, Fu Y, Shoham Z (2014) Double stimulations during the follicular and luteal phases of poor responders in IVF/ICSI programmes (Shanghai protocol). Reprod Biomed Online 29(6):684–691. doi:10.1016/j.rbmo.2014.08.009

Chapter 3
Embryo Cryopreservation in Breast Cancer Patients

Giuliano Bedoschi and Kutluk Oktay

Abstract Breast cancer is the second most common type of cancer expected to occur in women in 2014, accounting for 29 % of incident cases among women. Approximately 11 % of all breast cancer cases occur in women <45 years. Most of those patients are likely to undergo adjuvant systemic chemotherapy with a significant impact on ovarian reserve and future reproductive potential. Embryo cryopreservation is the most established technique for fertility preservation. This procedure is an attractive strategy for fertility preservation in reproductive age breast cancer patients with available partner or willing to use donor semen. Some special considerations should be given to ovarian stimulation for fertility preservation in breast cancer patients. The development of ovarian stimulation protocols using aromatase inhibitor combined with gonadotropin appears to be effective and safe for breast cancer patients. In this chapter, we will appraise and summarize the current state of embryo cryopreservation in breast cancer patients in order to provide a better understanding of the efficacy and safety of this fertility preservation technique.

Keywords Embryo cryopreservation • Breast cancer • Fertility preservation • Ovarian stimulation • Letrozole

3.1 Introduction

Breast cancer is a major public health problem in the United States and lives up to large investments in research, prevention, early diagnosis, and treatment.

Breast cancer is the second most common type of cancer expected to occur in women in 2014, accounting for 29 % (232,670) of incident cases among women [1]. The relatively stable incidence rates during the past 5 years for which there are data reflect improvements in cancer control and screening methods. At the same time, the detection of cancer at an early stage and the development of the treatment

G. Bedoschi • K. Oktay (✉)
New York Medical College, 40 Sunshine Cottage Rd, Valhalla, NY 10595, USA

Innovation Institute for Fertility Preservation and In Vitro Fertilization, New York, NY, USA
e-mail: koktay@fertilitypreservation.org

N. Suzuki, J. Donnez (eds.), *Gonadal Tissue Cryopreservation in Fertility Preservation*, DOI 10.1007/978-4-431-55963-4_3

modalities have contributed to improvements in survival over the past three decades, leading to an increase in the number of survivors [2]. Five-year relative survival rates for women has increased from 75 % for those diagnosed between 1975 and 1977 to 90 % for those diagnosed between 2003 and 2009 [1]. Moreover, recent estimates suggest that more than two million women living in the United States are currently survivors of breast cancer, making it the largest group of cancer survivors [3].

Approximately 11 % of all breast cancer cases occur in women <45 years [4]. As almost one quarter of first live births in the United States occur between the ages of 30 and 40, many of these women will have childbearing age [5]. Adjuvant chemotherapy is recommended for most patients with invasive disease in early stages, except for those with endocrine-sensitive tumors and with favorable prognostic features [6]. However, for unknown reasons, breast cancer in young women is associated with unfavorable prognostic features and higher recurrence rates compared with women diagnosed at an advanced age [7]. For these reasons, most women diagnosed with reproductive age in breast cancer will be treated with adjuvant chemotherapy, with a significant impact on ovarian reserve and future reproductive potential.

The impact of chemotherapy on ovarian reserve of women diagnosed with breast cancer is related to patient age, ovarian reserve, and chemotherapy regimen, particularly the doses of alkylating agents such as cyclophosphamide as these are known to be the most aggressive agents for ovarian reserve [8]. The patients of reproductive age diagnosed with breast cancer should be counseled about the possible risks of developing premature ovarian failure and infertility after chemotherapy [9]. Furthermore, as most of these patients present concerned with the impairment of reproductive potential after breast cancer treatment breast, fertility preservation became an increasingly important part of cancer care with attention to the improvement of post survival quality of life.

The available fertility preservation methods in breast cancer patients range from established fertility preservation techniques such as embryo and oocyte cryopreservation to experimental techniques such as ovarian tissue cryopreservation and cryopreservation of immature or in vitro matured oocytes. Moreover, the decision for the fertility preservation technique should consider the patient's age, type of treatment, diagnosis, whether she has a partner, and the time available for treatment. This chapter aims to update the knowledge about the use of embryo cryopreservation as a fertility preservation technique for breast cancer patients.

3.2 The Effect of Breast Cancer Treatment on Fertility

3.2.1 Ovarian Function Following Chemotherapy for Breast Cancer

Modern methods of cancer treatments have a significant negative impact on ovarian endocrine and reproductive function. The ovaries are adversely affected by multi-agent chemotherapy regimens, especially when alkylating agents are administered. Cyclophosphamide is an efficient alkylating agent as adjuvant treatment for breast cancer. However, it appears to have more toxic effects in the ovaries and therefore is associated with highest risk of infertility. Doxorubicin, cisplatin, and carboplatin are classified as medium-risk agents for gonadal dysfunction. The impact of taxanes on the primordial follicle population still remains unclear [8].

In women, the primordial follicles are nonrenewable, and their numbers are reduced throughout the female life span, until near-complete depletion prompts menopause. The majority of the follicles will be wasted due to apoptotic cell death during reproductive life [10]. The gonadotoxic chemotherapy agents facilitate the aging process in the ovaries, causing accelerated and premature depletion of primordial follicles [10, 11]. The predominant mechanism for the destruction of primordial follicles by chemotherapy has not been fully elucidated, although some studies suggested that direct toxic insults to the oocyte and to the surrounding steroid-producing somatic cell layers resulting in activation of apoptotic pathways are the main mechanism underlying gonadal failure [12, 13]. Individual patient features such as age and individual ovarian reserve may modulate the impact of a cancer treatment on the primordial follicle pool. Due to the reduction of the primordial follicle pool with aging, the risk of developing ovarian failure and infertility is higher in older women after a cytotoxic treatment compared with younger women. Consequently, depending on the age of the patient, ovarian failure may occur immediately or after chemotherapy prematurely [14].

3.2.2 Endocrine Therapy and Reproductive Function

In addition to chemotherapy, about two-thirds of premenopausal patients have hormone receptor-positive tumor and will receive tamoxifen for a period of 5–10 years, which has been shown to improve both recurrence-free and survival rates in this population [15, 16].

While it is commonly assumed that chemotherapy affects fertility, it is important to note that hormonal therapy has indirect effects and the delay of conception in order to receive several years of hormonal therapy may also affect the chance of successful conception.

First, tamoxifen has teratogenic effects [17] and thus should not be used during pregnancy [18]. Therefore, patients would have an increased risk of infertility, just for the reduction of the primordial follicle pool with aging. Second, tamoxifen may alter ovarian endocrine and reproductive function, resulting in fertility disorders, including an increased likelihood of amenorrhea [19].

3.3 Embryo Cryopreservation for Fertility Preservation

The first pregnancy resulting from transfer of a cryopreserved human embryo was reported in 1983 [20]. In the years since, advances in cryopreservation methods have made embryo cryopreservation the most established technique for fertility preservation. This procedure is an attractive strategy for fertility preservation in reproductive age breast cancer patients with available partner or willing to use donor semen. The process of embryo cryopreservation involves a sequence of highly coordinated steps beginning with controlled ovarian hyperstimulation (COH), followed by oocyte retrieval performed via transvaginal aspiration guided by ultrasonography under intravenous sedation, fertilization in the laboratory, and embryo cryopreservation [21]. The embryo transfer will be postponed until after the end of cancer treatment, when clearance for pregnancy has been obtained from the medical oncologist.

3.3.1 Ovarian Stimulation Protocols in Breast Cancer Patients

An in vitro fertilization (IVF) cycle typically requires 2–6 weeks to complete, depending on where in the menstrual cycle the patient presents. This time period may not be available to most cancer patients with the exception of women with breast cancer, who generally have a window of approximately 6–8 weeks between surgery and the initiation of adjuvant chemotherapy [22, 23].

Some special considerations should be given to ovarian stimulation for fertility preservation in breast cancer patients. First, the ideal ovarian stimulation regimen for fertility preservation in breast cancer patients should have a low risk of ovarian hyperstimulation syndrome (OHSS), as the majority of these patients will need to start chemotherapy shortly after oocyte retrieval [24, 25]. It is also important to reduce estrogen exposure during COH for fertility preservation, as higher hormonal levels may accelerate tumor growth in breast cancer [26]. In many circumstances, there may be insufficient time for traditional COH, and random-start protocols can be used with good results [27, 28].

3.3.1.1 GnRH Antagonist Protocol

Ovarian stimulation protocols using GnRH antagonist offer potential advantages over agonists, as the risk of OHSS appears lower when compared to agonist [29]. Furthermore, the use of antagonist provides the opportunity to use a GnRH agonist to trigger final oocyte maturation, thereby possibly further decreasing the risk of OHSS [24, 25]. The use of GnRH agonist trigger can also reduce the time interval from oocyte retrieval to the next menses, because of the suppressive effects that agonists may exert on ovarian response to gonadotropin stimulation [21]. This may help improve the feasibility of performing two consecutive ovarian stimulation cycles to increase the oocyte/embryo yield for fertility preservation before initiating cancer treatment [30].

3.3.1.2 Aromatase Inhibitor Protocol

Aromatase inhibitors can be effective in breast cancer patients who may benefit from safer protocols that reduce estrogen exposure. Letrozole is a selective and highly potent third-generation aromatase inhibitor, the enzyme that catalyzes the rate-limiting step in estrogen production [31]. It reduces estrogen production by inhibiting the conversion of androgens to estrogens, resulting in a compensatory release of the hypothalamic-pituitary axis from estrogen negative feedback and increase in gonadotropin secretion that stimulates ovarian follicular development [32].

Ovarian stimulation protocols using letrozole combined with gonadotropins have been used in fertility preservation through embryo or oocyte cryopreservation in women with hormone-sensitive tumors [26]. Evidence for the efficacy of this approach is accumulating rapidly. Studies exploring the use of ovarian stimulation protocols using letrozole combined with gonadotropins suggest that this approach produces comparable results to standard IVF protocols with reduced estrogen exposure [31].

3.3.1.3 Random-Start Ovarian Stimulation Protocol

Traditionally, COS is initiated at the beginning of the follicular phase; however, some patients may not be able to delay the initiation of cancer treatment. The development of random-start ovarian stimulation protocols provided a significant advantage for cancer patients by decreasing the total time for the IVF cycle, which can be successfully completed within 2 weeks regardless of menstrual cycle day at the time of initial presentation without compromising oocyte yield, oocyte maturity, and fertilization rates. The biological rationale for this intervention hinge on the perception that human ovarian follicles develop in coordinated waves within the menstrual cycle and hence starting ovarian stimulation randomly, including after ovulation, could be possible [32].

Starting the ovarian stimulation with recombinant follicle-stimulating hormone (rFSH) concomitantly to GnRH antagonist to downregulate luteinizing hormone (LH) secretion and initiate luteolysis may be useful for patients presenting in the luteal phase [27, 28]. Likewise, ovarian stimulation commenced in the late follicular phase may produce comparable results when compared to conventional ovarian stimulation [33, 34]. This allows cryopreservation of mature oocytes or embryos within a time frame acceptable in many cancer diseases. Nevertheless, aromatase inhibitors can be administered with random-start ovarian stimulation protocols to reduce estrogen production.

Additional clinical studies are needed to determine the efficacy of this strategy, mainly regarding the pregnancy and live birth rates from the use of cryopreserved embryos originated from random-start ovarian stimulation.

3.3.1.4 In Vitro Maturation

Oocyte maturation is a complex process that includes both nuclear and cytoplasmic maturation. Nuclear maturation mainly involves germinal vesicle breakdown, typically elicited by the LH surge at ovulation, followed by chromosome segregation and, finally, extrusion of the first polar body [35, 36]. Cytoplasmic maturation is more complex to define, but involves organelles that reorganize and store the mRNA, proteins, and transcription factors required for oocyte maturation, fertilization, and subsequent embryonic development [37].

In vitro maturation (IVM) describes the maturation of immature oocytes in culture after transvaginal oocyte retrieval. Immature oocytes can be harvested from unstimulated or primed cycles and fertilized following IVM. This could benefit women facing imminent oncological treatment who have insufficient time to undergo conventional ovarian stimulation, or women who prefer to avoid estrogen exposure; however, the results achieved thus far do not approach those of standard IVF. Implantation rates are lower than those expected with standard IVF, and this often necessitates the transfer of a larger number of embryos, which may increase the risk of multiple pregnancies. On the other hand, since a small percentage of oocytes retrieved during IVF are immature and typically discarded, these immature oocytes could be subjected to IVM to increase the oocyte and embryo yield in fertility preservation cycles [38].

3.3.1.5 Safety of Ovarian Stimulation in Breast Cancer Patients

Concerns about safety of performing ovarian stimulation in premenopausal breast cancer patients are reasonable and understandable. A short-term follow-up study demonstrated that breast cancer patients who have undergone ovarian stimulation using aromatase inhibitor combined with gonadotropins have not shown an increase in the risk of breast cancer recurrence, after a median follow-up of approximately 2 years [39]. Therefore, ovarian stimulation protocols using aromatase inhibitor combined with gonadotropin appear to be safe and effective for ovarian stimulation in fertility preservation cycles. Nevertheless, further studies are needed to determine whether this ovarian stimulation protocol has an impact on recurrence or survival, including a longer period of follow-up and a larger number of patients.

3.3.2 Cryopreservation Methods

The objective of cryopreservation is to maintain long-term viability after long-term storage. Liquid nitrogen (−196 °C) is the preferred environment for long-term storage. Embryos can be stored in liquid nitrogen for long periods of time without affecting the embryo survival rates or pregnancy outcomes [40].

Currently, there are two main methods used for embryo cryopreservation: slow freezing and vitrification. In both, cellular water is gradually replaced by cryoprotectants via osmosis by passage through increasing concentrations of the cryoprotectants. In the slow-freeze method, dehydrated embryos are sealed in plastic straws or vials, cooled at approximately −2 °C/min, manual seeded at around −7 °C to initiate extracellular ice formation in a controlled manner, further cooled at approximately −0.3 °C/min to temperatures below −30 °C, and then stored in liquid nitrogen (−196 °C). The first phase of the freezing process is rapid to prevent ice crystal formation (more likely to occur with gradual cooling) and the second phase more gradual [41]. In the vitrification method, all embryos are exposed to very high concentrations of cryoprotectants in very small volumes for very short periods of time, together with flash frozen by immersion into liquid nitrogen, creating a solid glass-like state [42]. Thawing is the reverse of the freezing process. Thawing involves the removal of the frozen straws or vials from liquid nitrogen and gradually removal of cryoprotectant through decreasing concentrations of the cryoprotectant, followed by an interval of culture before transfer.

Embryos can be cryopreserved efficiently at any stage, from pronuclear stage to blastocyst [43]. At each stage of development, laboratories tend to formulate inclusion criteria for selection of embryos to be considered for cryopreservation. These criteria are often stricter than the criteria used to consider an embryo to be suitable for fresh transfer and may differ widely between units.

The freezing-thawing protocols and the stage of embryo cryopreservation vary significantly between laboratories, and consensus is currently lacking on the best practice for embryo cryopreservation. Numerous studies have compared embryo thaw survival, implantation, and pregnancy rates between the two methods of cryopreservation. However, no superiority for the method of cryopreservation can be described in terms of post-thaw survival rate of embryos and pregnancy rates [44]. Furthermore, no randomized controlled trials are available that compare the success rates of embryo cryopreservation between embryos cryopreserved at different stages of development, and the optimum stage to cryopreserve embryos is still controversial [45].

3.3.3 *Frozen Embryo Transfer*

The endometrium cyclic change during a menstrual cycle is an essential part of achieving the receptive conditions for embryo implantation. Successful implantation requires a receptive endometrium that results from the postovulatory production of estrogen and progesterone by the corpus luteum. Endometrium receptivity toward the blastocyst is limited to days 6–10 after LH surge [46, 47]. The risk of implantation failure markedly increases if blastocyst approaches the endometrium after postovulatory day 10. Therefore, the synchronization between the stage of embryonic development and the endometrial environment is the most important factor influencing the implantation potential of frozen embryo transfers (FETs) [48–50].

Frozen embryos can be transferred in either a monitored natural menstrual cycle in women with normal ovulatory function or in artificial cycle in which endometrial development is carefully controlled by programmed sequential treatment with exogenous estrogen and progesterone, either with or without additional GnRH agonists. In both natural (days after ovulation) and artificial cycles (days of progesterone treatment), the time of transfer is synchronized with the stage of embryo development. No differences have been reported regarding pregnancy rates or live birth rates [51, 52] when comparing FET in natural cycles to artificial cycles [51, 52].

3.3.3.1 When Should Cryopreserved Embryos Be Transferred in Breast Cancer Survivors?

Some oncologists recommend that women successfully treated for breast cancer wait at least 2 years after diagnosis before attempting conception. This time is the most critical observation period, in which early recurrences may manifest [53, 54]. Nevertheless, the risk of recurrence is determined by many factors, including age at diagnosis, lymph node involvement, tumor stage, tumor biological characteristics, and hormone receptor status. Thus, the decision regarding when to attempt conception should be individualized, and these factors should be taken into consideration when counseling young patients about interval time between diagnosis and pregnancy.

Regarding patients with hormone-receptor-positive disease, it is important to remember that tamoxifen has teratogenic effects [17] and should not be used during pregnancy [18]. Therefore, it is reasonable to advise waiting at least 2 months after treatment completion before attempting conception [15, 55].

3.3.3.2 Endometrial Preparation for Frozen Embryo Transfer in Breast Cancer Survivors

In our center, breast cancer survivors are prepared for embryo transfer with an artificial cycle. First, preliminary downregulation with a GnRH agonist is initiated during the midluteal phase of previous menstrual cycle. After the onset of menses, endometrial development is carefully controlled by treatment with exogenous estrogen patches. Endometrial development is monitored until endometrial thickness reached >7 mm and a triple line pattern is evident on ultrasound examination. Once endometrial optimum characteristics are confirmed by ultrasound, progesterone is administered vaginally to support the luteal phase. Embryo transfer is performed 3–5 days later under transabdominal ultrasound guidance. Intramuscular progesterone is added for 7 days during the peri-implantation phase [56].

3.3.4 Frozen Embryo Transfer Outcomes in Breast Cancer Survivors

Overall, frozen embryo transfer has a reliable success rate. Even though pregnancy rates for frozen embryo transfer cycles in infertility patients are approximately two-thirds to those observed in fresh transfer cycles, this could be associated to an embryo selection bias due to highest quality embryos being selected during the fresh transfer. Results achieved with embryos frozen in cases of OHSS [57] as well as in cases of fertility preservation [56] appear to be similar to fresh transfer cycles.

The first and largest prospective study providing pregnancy outcome data from breast cancer patients undergoing frozen embryo transfer subsequent to ovarian stimulation was recently reported by our group [56]. In our experience, 33 patients diagnosed with $\leq$ stage 3 breast cancer underwent FET to themself or gestacional carrier (GC) with embryos generated from ovarian stimulation with letrozole-FSH protocol before adjuvant chemotherapy.

The patient's mean age at cryopreservation was 36.2 ± 4.2 years. Of the 33 women attempting pregnancy, 26 underwent FET once and 7 did twice, yielding 40 embryo transfers. Among these, 22 (55 %) were to a GC. Overall clinical pregnancy per FET, live birth per FET, and implantation rates were 65.0 % (26 out of 40), 45.0 % (18 out of 40), and 40.7 % (33 out of 81), respectively. From the total 18 pregnancies, 7 (38.8 %) were twins, with no higher-order pregnancies encountered.

Moreover, despite the fact that studies of the offspring resulting from IVF have raised concerns that the children may be at increased risk for obstetrical and perinatal outcomes [58, 59], our data did not show such an increase risk. Likewise, no fetal anomalies or malformation occurred and no developmental problems were reported by parents in a short-term follow-up.

The foregoing indicates that embryo cryopreservation with the letrozole-gonadotropin protocol yields success rates at least similar to those achieved with standard protocols used in general infertility populations and hence is highly successful in preserving fertility.

3.3.5 Gestational Surrogacy

Gestational surrogacy offers some breast cancer survivors the opportunity to have a genetic offspring. Gestational surrogacy involves transfer of embryos to the uterus of a woman willing to carry a pregnancy on behalf of a couple. Surrogacy is an option for breast cancer survivors with serious medical condition for which pregnancy may pose a life-threatening risk or for breast cancer survivors using medications that are, or could potentially be, teratogenic, such as tamoxifen.

The gestational carrier may be someone know or unknown to the couple who may or may not be compensated for her service. Candidates for surrogacy should have at least one, term, uncomplicated pregnancy and undergo thorough psychosocial evaluation and counseling by a qualified mental health professional. The legal issues of gestational surrogacy vary widely among different states, and even where it has recognition, a formal legal contract is required to formalize agreements between the infertile couple and the surrogate [60, 61].

3.4 Pregnancy Following Breast Cancer

There is little evidence to suggest that pregnancy adversely affects survival of women with a history of breast cancer. Retrospectives studies found no difference in rates of recurrences or distant metastases [54, 62]. Further studies have also compared the prognosis among patients with or without subsequent pregnancy and found that those women who attained pregnancy had superior survival compared with controls [63]. These data should be interpreted with caution as these studies included a small number of patients and have some methodological limitations. In our experience, we observed no breast cancer recurrences after pregnancy among women undergoing FET to their own uterus after a median follow-up of approximately 3 years [56].

No data suggest that lactation increases the risk of breast cancer recurrence. Successful lactation and breastfeeding are possible depending on the degree of surgical intervention and radiation exposure, even from the treated side [64].

3.5 Summary and Conclusion

Breast cancer is a common disease among women and frequently affects premenopausal women. Most of those patients are likely to undergo adjuvant systemic chemotherapy with recognized gonadotoxic effects. In addition to this, women with hormone-sensitive tumors will receive a 5–10 years course of adjuvant hormonal therapy with tamoxifen during which time pregnancy is not allowed. This delay will further reduce the chances of latter successful pregnancy mainly by ovarian aging. Embryo cryopreservation is the most established technique for fertility preservation, which involves deep freeze of an embryo. The procedure can be offered to premenopausal women diagnosed with breast cancer with available partner or willing to use donor semen. At the time of desired pregnancy, the embryo is thawed and transferred to the uterus. However, concerns with estrogen exposure and timing requirements for this procedure currently limit the feasibility for many breast cancer patients. The development of ovarian stimulation protocols using aromatase inhibitor combined with gonadotropin appears to be effective and safe for breast cancer patients. Further improvements in letrozole-gonadotropin protocol have been reported. Triggering oocyte maturation with GnRH agonist resulted in improvement in outcomes by increasing the yield of mature oocytes and embryos, as well as decreasing estradiol exposure after trigger, and reducing the risk of ovarian hyperstimulation syndrome in women with breast cancer. The earlier in the process the women receives fertility counseling, the greater the number of fertility preservation options that are likely to be available without compromise in prognosis.

References

1. Siegel R, Ma J, Zou Z, Jemal A (2014) Cancer statistics, 2014. CA Cancer J Clin 64(1):9–29
2. DeSantis C, Siegel R, Bandi P, Jemal A (2011) Breast cancer statistics, 2011. CA Cancer J Clin 61(6):409–418
3. Ganz PA, Hahn EE (2008) Implementing a survivorship care plan for patients with breast cancer. J Clin Oncol 26(5):759–767
4. Trivers KF, Fink AK, Partridge AH et al (2014) Estimates of young breast cancer survivors at risk for infertility in the U.S. Oncologist 19(8):814–822
5. Hayat MJ, Howlader N, Reichman ME, Edwards BK (2007) Cancer statistics, trends, and multiple primary cancer analyses from the Surveillance, Epidemiology, and End Results (SEER) Program. Oncologist 12(1):20–37
6. Goldhirsch A, Wood WC, Gelber RD et al (2007) Progress and promise: highlights of the international expert consensus on the primary therapy of early breast cancer 2007. Ann Oncol 18(7):1133–1144
7. Anders CK, Hsu DS, Broadwater G et al (2008) Young age at diagnosis correlates with worse prognosis and defines a subset of breast cancers with shared patterns of gene expression. J Clin Oncol 26(20):3324–3330

8. Loren AW, Mangu PB, Beck LN et al (2013) Fertility preservation for patients with cancer: American Society of Clinical Oncology clinical practice guideline update. J Clin Oncol 31(19):2500–2510
9. Partridge AH, Gelber S, Peppercorn J et al (2004) Web-based survey of fertility issues in young women with breast cancer. J Clin Oncol 22(20):4174–4183
10. Gosden RG, Faddy MJ (1994) Ovarian aging, follicular depletion, and steroidogenesis. Exp Gerontol 29(3–4):265–274
11. Meirow D, Nugent D (2001) The effects of radiotherapy and chemotherapy on female reproduction. Hum Reprod Update 7(6):535–543
12. Tilly JL, Kolesnick RN (2002) Sphingolipids, apoptosis, cancer treatments and the ovary: investigating a crime against female fertility. Biochim Biophys Acta 1585(2–3):135–138
13. Soleimani R, Heytens E, Darzynkiewicz Z, Oktay K (2011) Mechanisms of chemotherapy-induced human ovarian aging: double strand DNA breaks and microvascular compromise. Aging 3(8):782–793
14. Byrne J, Fears TR, Gail MH et al (1992) Early menopause in long-term survivors of cancer during adolescence. Am J Obstet Gynecol 166(3):788–793
15. Davies C, Pan H, Godwin J et al (2013) Long-term effects of continuing adjuvant tamoxifen to 10 years versus stopping at 5 years after diagnosis of oestrogen receptor-positive breast cancer: ATLAS, a randomised trial. Lancet 381(9869):805–816
16. Early Breast Cancer Trialists' Collaborative G (2005) Effects of chemotherapy and hormonal therapy for early breast cancer on recurrence and 15-year survival: an overview of the randomised trials. Lancet 365(9472):1687–1717
17. Braems G, Denys H, De Wever O, Cocquyt V, Van den Broecke R (2011) Use of tamoxifen before and during pregnancy. Oncologist 16(11):1547–1551
18. Ruddy KJ, Partridge AH (2012) The unique reproductive concerns of young women with breast cancer. Adv Exp Med Biol 732:77–87
19. Hulvat MC, Jeruss JS (2011) Fertility preservation options for young women with breast cancer. Curr Opin Obstet Gynecol 23(3):174–182
20. Trounson A, Mohr L (1983) Human pregnancy following cryopreservation, thawing and transfer of an eight-cell embryo. Nature 305(5936):707–709
21. Bedoschi G, Oktay K (2013) Current approach to fertility preservation by embryo cryopreservation. Fertil Steril 99(6):1496–1502
22. Baynosa J, Westphal LM, Madrigrano A, Wapnir I (2009) Timing of breast cancer treatments with oocyte retrieval and embryo cryopreservation. J Am Coll Surg 209(5):603–607
23. Madrigrano A, Westphal L, Wapnir I (2007) Egg retrieval with cryopreservation does not delay breast cancer treatment. Am J Surg 194(4):477–481
24. Oktay K, Turkcuoglu I, Rodriguez-Wallberg KA (2010) GnRH agonist trigger for women with breast cancer undergoing fertility preservation by aromatase inhibitor/FSH stimulation. Reprod Biomed Online 20(6):783–788
25. Reddy J, Turan V, Bedoschi G, Moy F, Oktay K (2014) Triggering final oocyte maturation with gonadotropin-releasing hormone agonist (GnRHa) versus human chorionic gonadotropin (hCG) in breast cancer patients undergoing fertility preservation: an extended experience. J Assist Reprod Genet 31(7):927–932
26. Reddy J, Oktay K (2012) Ovarian stimulation and fertility preservation with the use of aromatase inhibitors in women with breast cancer. Fertil Steril 98(6):1363–1369
27. von Wolff M, Thaler CJ, Frambach T et al (2009) Ovarian stimulation to cryopreserve fertilized oocytes in cancer patients can be started in the luteal phase. Fertil Steril 92(4): 1360–1365
28. Bedoschi GM, de Albuquerque FO, Ferriani RA, Navarro PA (2010) Ovarian stimulation during the luteal phase for fertility preservation of cancer patients: case reports and review of the literature. J Assist Reprod Genet 27(8):491–494
29. von Wolff M, Montag M, Dittrich R, Denschlag D, Nawroth F, Lawrenz B (2011) Fertility preservation in women – a practical guide to preservation techniques and therapeutic strategies

in breast cancer, Hodgkin's lymphoma and borderline ovarian tumours by the fertility preservation network FertiPROTEKT. Arch Gynecol Obstet 284(2):427–435
30. Turan V, Bedoschi G, Moy F, Oktay K (2013) Safety and feasibility of performing two consecutive ovarian stimulation cycles with the use of letrozole-gonadotropin protocol for fertility preservation in breast cancer patients. Fertil Steril 100(6):1681–1685, e1681
31. Oktay K, Hourvitz A, Sahin G et al (2006) Letrozole reduces estrogen and gonadotropin exposure in women with breast cancer undergoing ovarian stimulation before chemotherapy. J Clin Endocrinol Metab 91(10):3885–3890
32. Baerwald AR, Adams GP, Pierson RA (2003) A new model for ovarian follicular development during the human menstrual cycle. Fertil Steril 80(1):116–122
33. Sonmezer M, Turkcuoglu I, Coskun U, Oktay K (2011) Random-start controlled ovarian hyperstimulation for emergency fertility preservation in letrozole cycles. Fertil Steril 95(6): 2125 e2129–2111
34. Cakmak H, Rosen MP (2013) Ovarian stimulation in cancer patients. Fertil Steril 99(6): 1476–1484
35. Memili E, Peddinti D, Shack LA et al (2007) Bovine germinal vesicle oocyte and cumulus cell proteomics. Reproduction 133(6):1107–1120
36. Tatemoto H, Muto N, Sunagawa I, Shinjo A, Nakada T (2004) Protection of porcine oocytes against cell damage caused by oxidative stress during in vitro maturation: role of superoxide dismutase activity in porcine follicular fluid. Biol Reprod 71(4):1150–1157
37. Watson AJ (2007) Oocyte cytoplasmic maturation: a key mediator of oocyte and embryo developmental competence. J Anim Sci 85(13 Suppl):E1–E3
38. Oktay K, Buyuk E, Rodriguez-Wallberg KA, Sahin G (2010) In vitro maturation improves oocyte or embryo cryopreservation outcome in breast cancer patients undergoing ovarian stimulation for fertility preservation. Reprod Biomed Online 20(5):634–638
39. Azim AA, Costantini-Ferrando M, Oktay K (2008) Safety of fertility preservation by ovarian stimulation with letrozole and gonadotropins in patients with breast cancer: a prospective controlled study. J Clin Oncol 26(16):2630–2635
40. Wirleitner B, Vanderzwalmen P, Bach M et al (2013) The time aspect in storing vitrified blastocysts: its impact on survival rate, implantation potential and babies born. Hum Reprod 28(11):2950–2957
41. Wong KM, Mastenbroek S, Repping S (2014) Cryopreservation of human embryos and its contribution to in vitro fertilization success rates. Fertil Steril 102(1):19–26
42. Herrero L, Martinez M, Garcia-Velasco JA (2011) Current status of human oocyte and embryo cryopreservation. Curr Opin Obstet Gynecol 23(4):245–250
43. Edgar DH, Gook DA (2012) A critical appraisal of cryopreservation (slow cooling versus vitrification) of human oocytes and embryos. Hum Reprod Update 18(5):536–554
44. Loutradi KE, Kolibianakis EM, Venetis CA et al (2008) Cryopreservation of human embryos by vitrification or slow freezing: a systematic review and meta-analysis. Fertil Steril 90(1): 186–193
45. Glujovsky D, Blake D, Farquhar C, Bardach A (2012) Cleavage stage versus blastocyst stage embryo transfer in assisted reproductive technology. Cochrane Database Syst Rev 7: CD002118
46. Paulson RJ (2011) Hormonal induction of endometrial receptivity. Fertil Steril 96(3):530–535
47. Wilcox AJ, Baird DD, Weinberg CR (1999) Time of implantation of the conceptus and loss of pregnancy. N Engl J Med 340(23):1796–1799
48. Cha J, Sun X, Dey SK (2012) Mechanisms of implantation: strategies for successful pregnancy. Nat Med 18(12):1754–1767
49. Norwitz ER, Schust DJ, Fisher SJ (2001) Implantation and the survival of early pregnancy. N Engl J Med 345(19):1400–1408
50. Quenby S, Brosens JJ (2013) Human implantation: a tale of mutual maternal and fetal attraction. Biol Reprod 88(3):81

51. Ghobara T, Vandekerckhove P (2008) Cycle regimens for frozen-thawed embryo transfer. Cochrane Database Syst Rev 1:CD003414
52. Groenewoud ER, Cantineau AE, Kollen BJ, Macklon NS, Cohlen BJ (2013) What is the optimal means of preparing the endometrium in frozen-thawed embryo transfer cycles? A systematic review and meta-analysis. Hum Reprod Update 19(5):458–470
53. Ives A, Saunders C, Bulsara M, Semmens J (2007) Pregnancy after breast cancer: population based study. BMJ 334(7586):194
54. Petrek JA (1994) Pregnancy safety after breast cancer. Cancer 74(1 Suppl):528–531
55. Azim HA Jr, Peccatori FA, de Azambuja E, Piccart MJ (2011) Motherhood after breast cancer: searching for la dolce vita. Expert Rev Anticancer Ther 11(2):287–298
56. Oktay KTV, Bedoschi G, Pacheco F, Moy F (2015) Fertility preservation success subsequent to concurrent aromatase inhibitor treatment and ovarian stimulation in women with breast cancer. J Clin Oncol 33(22):2424–2429
57. D'Angelo A, Amso N (2007) Embryo freezing for preventing ovarian hyperstimulation syndrome. Cochrane Database Syst Rev 3:CD002806
58. Helmerhorst FM, Perquin DA, Donker D, Keirse MJ (2004) Perinatal outcome of singletons and twins after assisted conception: a systematic review of controlled studies. BMJ 328(7434): 261
59. Henningsen AK, Pinborg A, Lidegaard O, Vestergaard C, Forman JL, Andersen AN (2011) Perinatal outcome of singleton siblings born after assisted reproductive technology and spontaneous conception: Danish national sibling-cohort study. Fertil Steril 95(3):959–963
60. Practice Committee of the American Society for Reproductive M, Practice Committee of the Society for Assisted Reproductive T (2015) Recommendations for practices utilizing gestational carriers: a committee opinion. Fertil Steril 103(1):e1–e8
61. Dar S, Lazer T, Swanson S et al (2015) Assisted reproduction involving gestational surrogacy: an analysis of the medical, psychosocial and legal issues: experience from a large surrogacy program. Hum Reprod 30(2):345–352
62. Surbone A, Petrek JA (1997) Childbearing issues in breast carcinoma survivors. Cancer 79(7): 1271–1278
63. Gelber S, Coates AS, Goldhirsch A et al (2001) Effect of pregnancy on overall survival after the diagnosis of early-stage breast cancer. J Clin Oncology 19(6):1671–1675
64. Higgins S, Haffty BG (1994) Pregnancy and lactation after breast-conserving therapy for early stage breast cancer. Cancer 73(8):2175–2180

Chapter 4
Ovarian Tissue Cryopreservation: Slow Freezing

Sonia Herraiz, Cesar Diaz-Garcia, and Antonio Pellicer

Abstract The needs for fertility preservation (FP) have substantially increased due to improvements in early diagnosis and survival of many malignancies experienced during the last decades. Different FP options can be offered nowadays, but ovarian tissue cryopreservation and retransplantation is the preferred option in prepubertal girls or when there is an urgent need to start the treatment (no time for ovarian stimulation). In this chapter, the basic principles of cryopreservation will be reviewed. A comprehensive and clinical practice-oriented description of the retrieval, preparation, and slow-freezing procedure of the tissue will be provided, together with a summary of the cryopreservation protocols that have been proven to be effective by obtaining live births.

Keywords Cancer • Cryopreservation • Fertility • Ovary

4.1 Introduction

The improvements achieved in the field of oncology during the last two decades had completely changed the management and priorities of the patients. The combined 5 years relative survival rate for children with cancer, including all cancer sites, has improved from around 63 to 79 % in the last 20 years [1]. Despite this increase in survival rates, current regimens of multi-agent chemotherapy and radiotherapy cause numerous side effects, one of them being infertility. This implies that a

S. Herraiz • A. Pellicer
Reproductive Medicine Research Group, IIS La Fe. La Fe University Hospital, Valencia, Spain

IVI Foundation, Valencia, Spain

Department of Pediatrics, Obstetrics and Gynecology, University of Valencia, Valencia, Spain

C. Diaz-Garcia (✉)
Reproductive Medicine Research Group, IIS La Fe. La Fe University Hospital, Valencia, Spain

Department of Pediatrics, Obstetrics and Gynecology, University of Valencia, Valencia, Spain
e-mail: cesar.diaz@uv.es

N. Suzuki, J. Donnez (eds.), *Gonadal Tissue Cryopreservation in Fertility Preservation*, DOI 10.1007/978-4-431-55963-4_4

growing number of pediatric patients will reach the reproductive age and will experience the side effect of cancer treatments. It is also important to highlight that the most common malignancy during the reproductive age in women is breast cancer and that 6.4 % of patients are younger than 40 years old [2]. Survival rates in this population have increased from 74.9 % in the mid-1970s to 87.7 % in the late 1990s [3]. In summary, around 8 % of all cancer patients are less than 40 years of age [4], and around 0.4 % of all young women are cancer survivors with this proportion rising in the future [5].

The degree of gonadotoxicity varies between the different groups of chemotherapeutic drugs; in general, alkylating agents are those at higher risk of gonadotoxicity [6]. For example, in a study carried out in patients with Hodgkin's lymphoma, it was found that the 10-year probabilities of achieving parenthood were 55 % after use of chemotherapy considered to be of low gonadotoxicity, 51 % after use of chemotherapy considered to be of medium gonadotoxicity, and 27 % after use of chemotherapy considered to be of high gonadotoxicity [7].

The mechanism by which the chemotherapeutic agents compromise the ovary is the loss of a large number of follicles of various stages, including the pool of primordial follicles, causing a decrease in overall ovarian size [8]. Such effect is usually caused by induction of apoptosis, but also through uncontrolled activation of primordial follicles [9], which motivates a burnout of the primordial follicle pool. Chemotherapy can also induce injury to blood vessels and focal fibrosis of the ovarian cortex [6].

The ovarian toxicity of chemotherapeutic agents is largely dependent on the patient's age [10]. A recent large study of posttreatment parenthood in patients with Hodgkin's lymphoma [7] showed that the probability for parenthood 15 years after treatment was different in women younger than 30 years of age at diagnosis (85–89 %) than in those older than 30 years (25 %).

Concerning the ovarian toxicity of radiotherapy, the damage to the ovaries is dependent on the dose of radiation over the ovaries [11], and fractionation of the dose makes it less harmful than a single dose. The oocyte is a type of cell that is very sensitive to radiation, and it has been estimated that a low dose of 2–4 Gy over the ovaries destroys around half of the oocytes [12]. Several of the radiation protocols that are used nowadays include radiation doses up to 40 and 50 Gy, for example, those used for primary or adjuvant treatment of advanced cervical cancer [13] and rectal cancer [14], total-body irradiation in preparation for allogenic hematopoietic stem cell transplantation [15], and as co-treatment together with chemotherapy for lymphoma [16], Ewing's sarcoma [17], or Wilms' tumor [18, 19].

Beside the oncologic patients, there is another group of patients suffering from nonmalignant diseases whose evolution will require aggressive therapeutic interventions such as a BMT or severe immunosuppression induced by chemotherapeutic agents. This group of patients with pathologies such as thalassemia, drepanocytosis, demyelinating diseases, lupus, or genetic disorders whose treatments will compromise the ovarian function, can represent close to 20 % of the patients undergoing a fertility preservation (FP) procedure in some series [20].

Different available options exist to keep the reproductive function after the use of gonadotoxic treatments, such as controlled ovarian stimulation (COS) to preserve oocytes and embryos, in vitro maturation of immature oocytes (IVM), pituitary downregulation to induce quiescence of the ovary, or ovarian tissue cryopreservation. Embryo and oocyte cryopreservation are recognized by the ASRM as the only established methods for FP [21]. Despite new rapid COS protocols starting stimulation irrespective of the stage of the menstrual cycle, it takes around 11 days to collect mature oocytes suitable for IVF or vitrification [22] (see Chaps. 2, 3 and 4 for extended information). IVM can help to improve the pool of vitrified mature oocytes when used together with other techniques [23], but its efficiency is quite poor when used alone in normo-ovulatory women [24]. Ovarian tissue cryopreservation has been suggested as the preferred method for FP in prepubertal females in whom COS is not feasible and in situations in which the beginning of the gonadotoxic treatment cannot be delayed. Ovarian cortex retrieval can be done even on the same day of the first consultation, and chemotherapy can start almost immediately after if needed, causing virtually no delay in oncologic treatments.

4.2 Principles of Cryopreservation

The main goal of the cryopreservation procedure is to minimize tissue injury from low, subzero temperatures [25]. The storage at a low temperature can stop the biological clock for an unlimited time [26]. This is due to the fact that very low temperatures virtually stop any chemical reaction and increase collision time between molecules, avoiding tissue degradation at a molecular level (DNA, protein, or lipidic degradation). Nevertheless, by lowering the temperature of a living cell, ice crystals can be formed from liquid water, increasing the intracellular volume and breaking cell membranes, causing cell death. Therefore, the objective of cryopreservation is to allow temperatures low enough to stop biochemical reactions and avoid/minimize ice crystal formation inside the cells.

4.2.1 Ice Formation

The main constituent of any cell is water, which makes up to 60–85 % of the cell volume [27]. Cells contain "free" water and "bound" water (Fig. 4.1). The bound water is essential to maintain cell structure and function, and they are incapable of freezing [28] as long as they remain attached to other molecules. Thus, water plays an important role in cryobiology since at cooling to low subzero temperature, 90 % of water in a cell will convert into ice (free water) [27] and the 10 % will not (some of the bound water will stay). The highest temperature when ice can form at normal

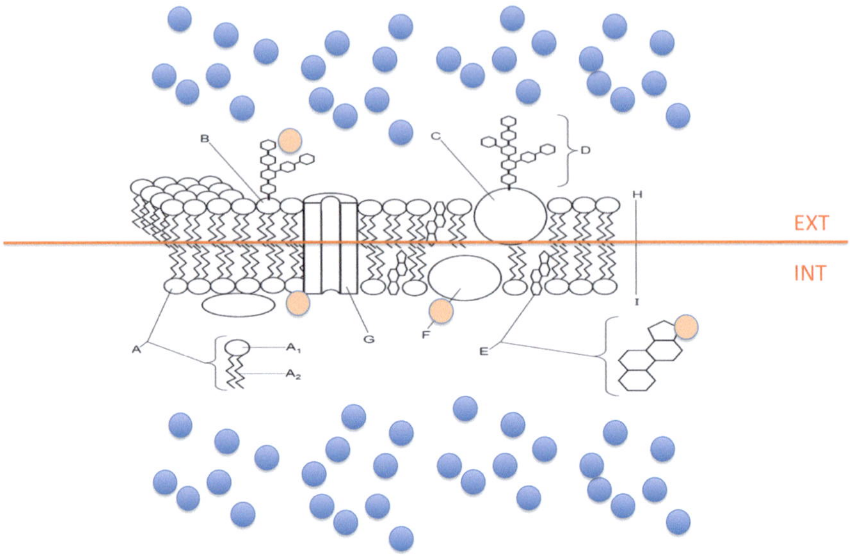

Fig. 4.1 Free water does not interact with other molecules (*blue circles* represent free water molecules: *1* oxygen atom and *2* hydrogen atoms), and bound water sticks to proteins, nucleic acids, and head groups of membrane phospholipids through hydrogen bridges (*brown circles* represent bound water). *INT* internal interface of the cell membrane, *EXT* external interface of the cell membrane

pressure is 0 °C. However, ice in general forms at temperatures between −5 and −15 °C because the formation of ice crystals releases heat [25].

4.2.2 *Cryoprotectants*

There are substances known as cryoprotectants (CPAs) whose function is to modify the formation and growth of ice. CPAs exist in nature in the form of sugars (sucrose, glucose, trehalose), small molecules (urea), and large proteins (antifreeze proteins superfamily). The CPAs can be divided into two categories:

4.2.2.1 Permeable Cryoprotectants

Permeable CPAs are small, nonionic molecules with low toxicity and high solubility in water. The rate of CPA permeation and dilution is determined by the species, cell type and stage of development, solution composition, temperature, and hydrostatic pressure [29]. The most commonly used permeable CPAs are dimethyl sulfoxide (DMSO), propylene glycol (PROH), and ethylene glycol (EG). The mechanisms by which these permeable CPAs protect living cells seem to be by lowering the freezing point by disrupting interactions between water molecules involved in ice crystal formation and also by stabilizing proteins and deoxyribonucleic acid. By avoiding ice formation, free water is more available; hence they also help to diminish the relative concentration of different solutes in the cell, minimizing osmotic changes. It has to be pointed out that at high concentrations, these substances can be detrimental to the cell survival due to the conformational changes induced in bigger molecules by hydrogen interaction.

4.2.2.2 Non-permeable Cryoprotectants

Non-permeable CPAs are usually long-chain molecules that do not cross the cell membrane; they are soluble in water and they increase the osmolality of the solution. The most frequently used non-permeable CPAs are disaccharides (sucrose, glucose, fructose, sorbitol, saccharose, trehalose), some macromolecules (polyvinilpyrrolidone (PVP), polyvinyl alcohol, Ficoll), and proteins (bovine serum albumin, BSA). They contribute to cell dehydration, thus avoiding ice crystal formation inside the cell by decreasing the availability of free water. They also counteract osmotic stress and reduce the toxicity of permeable CPAs [30].

4.2.3 Cryopreservation Procedures

There are two principally different cryopreservation procedures, slow freezing and vitrification. Both procedures include four common steps: exposure of the samples to CPA, freezing/cooling to the storage temperature (−196 °C), thawing/warming, and CPA removal. The main difference between these methods lays in the different cooling rates (cooling rates are around 30,000 times faster in vitrification than in slow freezing) and the mechanisms that will protect the cell against ice crystal formation (while in slow freezing ice crystal formation is driven to the extracellular space, in vitrification ice crystal formation is avoided by inducing a glass transition temperature higher than that of the freezing temperature, so that the water will become glass instead of ice).

4.2.3.1 Slow Freezing

Slow freezing is a method that aims at achieving the optimal balance (equilibrium) between the rates of cell dehydration and extracellular ice formation [31]. In this procedure, the CPA is added to the solution around the cells/tissue, and the cooling rate is dependent on the size and permeability of the specific cells/tissue to be cryopreserved. The slow-freezing method reduces the likelihood of intracellular ice formation by initiation of extracellular ice crystal formation (seeding) at a high subzero temperature (e.g., −6 to −9 °C). The extracellular ice draws water out of the cell until little amount of free water remains and only small (non-lethal) ice crystals have been formed [32]. The best outcome of this cryopreservation method is obtained when the rate of freezing allows equilibrium between the rate of water loss from the cell (dehydration) and the rate at which water is integrated into extracellular ice crystals. It should be pointed out that ice formation is an integral part of the slow-freezing procedure, but always in the extracellular matrix. The freezing rate differs between various cell types, and it is influenced by factors such as cell size, cell membrane permeability, and diffusion characteristics. The optimal cooling rate varies between 0.3 and 1 °C/min for oocytes and embryos [33], between 0.3 and 10 °C/min for ovarian tissue [34], and up to >1,000 °C/min for red blood cells [27]. The slow cooling procedure usually ends when the temperature lies between −30 and −80 °C and after that, the sample can be plunged into liquid nitrogen [25].

4.2.3.2 Vitrification

Vitrification is the procedure when a solution solidifies in a glass-like or vitreous state without any formation of ice crystals during cooling and remains in this state throughout the warming [25]. Vitrification involves the use of high concentrations of CPA, which interact strongly with water. These interactions avoid other interactions between water molecules, and this phenomenon subsequently avoids ice crystals formation. In order to cause such effect, CPA must penetrate the cells before cooling starts, and dehydration of the cells occur also before cooling which normally occurs very quickly (>20,000 °C/min) since the samples are usually plunged directly into liquid nitrogen (−196 °C) [25].

4.2.3.3 Thawing/Warming

The thawing and CPA removal are also important steps for a successful procedure. Cells cooled by slow freezing always contain some water, and proper thawing is essential to avoid ice damage [32]. There is an opinion that the ice formed during thawing is less dangerous [35], although some authors brought up the subject that slow thawing may be detrimental to the cells due to ice formation [36]. Regardless of the cryopreservation technique, the thawing procedure usually involves the passage through decreasing concentrations of CPA diluted in warm media.

4.2.4 Cryoinjury

Both freezing and thawing can cause cell damage, despite the use of CPA. This is known as cryoinjury and can be due to mechanic stress caused by ice formation inside or outside the cell, osmotic changes following dehydration, and rehydration involving the loss of bound water or even due to the use of CPA. However, decreasing the time and temperature of cell exposure to CPAs can reduce their toxicity, while stepwise addition and removal of CPAs decrease osmotic stress and excessive volume change of the cells [37]. It should be pointed out that the exact mechanism of cell damage during cryopreservation and CPA toxicity has not yet been elucidated [38, 39] although different mechanisms such as conformational changes in proteins, structural changes in lipidic bilayers, altered ion channel permeability, formation of toxic molecules inside the cell, or even DNA degradation (specially with the use of DMSO) have been suggested [38, 40].

Intracellular ice formation can occur when a cell is unable to maintain equilibrium with the extracellular space during slow freezing or when the critical cooling rate is not obtained by vitrification methods. If large crystals are formed in the extracellular space, cells can also be damaged from the outside [41, 42]. When vitrification and warming are done, a phenomenon known as devitrification results in recrystallization [43], that is, a formation of ice crystals during warming.

4.2.5 Histological Considerations of the Ovary Regarding Cryopreservation

The main ovarian functions are differentiation and release of mature oocyte competent for fertilization and production of steroid hormones necessary for secondary sexual characteristics, achievement, and early maintenance of pregnancy. According to Gougeon morphological classification [44], the different stages of maturation of the follicles are primordial follicles (the earliest stage) containing an oocyte surrounded by a single layer of flattened granulosa cells; primary follicles, surrounded by a single cuboidal layer of granulosa cells; secondary follicles, with more than one layer of cuboidal granulosa cells and theca externa and interna cells which originate from ovarian stroma; and antral follicles, when a fluid-filled antrum appears inside the granulosa cells. From primary follicles and beyond, the number of follicles decreases, the size increases, and the presence of higher amounts of water (antral follicles) makes them more difficult to cryopreserve.

4.2.5.1 Primordial Follicles

Primordial follicles are the main component of the ovarian reserve, representing up to 80 % of the follicular population [45]. They are characterized by their relative abundance and lack of differentiation: they measure less than 30 μm because they only have a monolayer of flat granulosa cells and the oocyte contained into them only has few organelles, lacks zona pellucida, and is metabolically quiescent and undifferentiated. These characteristics, particularly their small size, result in an increased resistance to freezing and thawing processes. Due to these properties, the primordial follicle population is an ideal choice for potential use in FP programs [46, 47].

In humans, the female germ cell population is formed before birth, and it is not substantially replenished during adult life [48]. It is also accepted that the fate of almost all of these germ cells is death [49–51]. Each human ovary contains ≈400,000 quiescent primordial follicles, and intraovarian mechanisms activate a small wave of them (≈1000/month) to initiate growth. Ovarian senescence and cessation of ovarian function occur during menopause, when less than 1000 follicles remain [52]. There is a wide variation between women in the number and rate of follicular depletion. Each quiescent follicle maintains the ability to begin its development and to reach advanced maturation stages and be ovulated or undergo atresia [53]; primordial follicles may also die directly from its dormant stage [49]. Several studies have been performed to elucidate the molecular mechanisms that control primordial follicle activation, but the underlying mechanisms of activation remain unknown.

4.2.5.2 Follicular Distribution Within the Ovary

The distribution of follicles is extremely uneven in ovarian tissue as pointed out by Lass, who carefully reviewed the previous published studies that considered the issue of follicular distribution and dynamics in the ovarian cortex through reproductive lifespan [54]. In a very illustrative experiment carried out in 24 patients, Qu and colleagues demonstrated such variability [45] showing a discrepancy between follicular densities in paired samples obtained from different sites of the same ovary.

The same erratic pattern was detected in other studies with independence of the diagnosis of the included patients. Thus, Kohl et al. [55] compared samples of the contralateral ovaries from five infertile women and biopsies from different sites of the same ovary; and Poirot et al. [56] collected ovarian tissue from 31 patients having chemotherapy. Both found large variation between the ovaries and between the sites of the biopsies. Another good example of this heterogeneity was provided by Schmidt et al. [57]; they found densities ranging from 1.1 to 190.6 follicles/mm^3 when examining ovarian biopsies from 21 oncologic patients. In all cases, a significant inverse correlation between follicular density and age was observed.

In adult women, primordial follicles are always located within the dense stroma of the ovarian cortex, while populations of primary or secondary follicles can be also at the corticomedullary junction or even in the medullar zone beneath the cortex [45]. In prepubertal girls, primordial follicles can also be found in great numbers in the medulla, especially in patients up to the age of 3–10 years old [58]. Then, the number of primordial follicles in the medulla decreases with age, and they experience a 17-fold decrease in the group of women aged 20–30 and around 55-fold decrease in the group of patients above 30 years old [58]. A vascular network involved in the control of the follicular development mechanisms is located surrounding the pre-antral follicle [59]. This vascular network transports signals to the granulosa cells, and the signal from the stimulated granulosa cells then reaches the oocytes through gap junctions. Simultaneously, angiogenesis in the ovarian medulla is necessary for the selective growth of the cortical follicles [60]. The mesenchymal cortex surrounding the follicles of the embryo and newborn is soft, while in adult ovaries accumulated collagen fibers transform the connective tissue, making it harder and less permeable. It is postulated that the characteristics of the environment surrounding the follicle, such as the density of vascular network and the softness of the interstitial tissue, determines the initiation of follicle growth. Taking into account all the abovementioned, the ovarian tissue preparation procedure, prior to cryopreservation, should guarantee that the selected fragment is composed by the outer part of the ovarian cortex (1 mm of thickness) in all cases.

4.3 Practical Tips for Ovarian Tissue Cryopreservation

4.3.1 Ovarian Tissue Retrieval

Ovarian tissue retrieval can be done through conventional laparoscopy, single site laparoscopy, or mini-laparotomy. Regardless of the surgical approach, the common aim is to provide an easy, fast, and harmless access to the tissue so that the patient can start her oncological treatment without any kind of delay. Most of the programs use the laparoscopic approach to harvest the ovarian tissue. Surgical times do not usually last for more than 30 min; the estimated blood loss and perioperative complications are virtually inexistent [61]. When performed in a day-surgery basis, the patients can be discharged in 6 h, without any kind of repercussion in terms of quality of life [61]. The mini-laparotomy approach is usually reserved for specific cases such as pediatric patients [62], although it can also be performed in adults [63]. In our series, we keep the mini-laparotomy approach exclusively for patients with a formal contraindication for general anesthesia. This group of patients is mainly represented by those with big mediastinal masses compromising the respiratory tract. In such cases, a spinal anesthesia and mini-laparotomy are performed.

Another important issue is the amount of tissue to be harvested. There is no consensus about the ideal amount. Nevertheless, there are some factors that could influence the decision on the amount to some extent:

1. The risk of ovarian failure after oncologic treatment: For very high risk treatments such as total-body irradiation or conditioning regimens with melphalan or busulfan, if the ovary is left in place, it is very likely that it will be completely damaged; therefore, an oophorectomy is preferred. It has to be pointed out that even “not-so-aggressive” regimens could compromise the ovarian function in patients with a potentially compromised ovarian reserve (e.g., women over 35 years old).

2. The quantity of primordial follicles contained in the tissue: this is a key determinant of the graft longevity and functionality [64]. Taking into account that we cannot modify the density of primordial follicles of a given patient, the simplest way to retrieve more follicles is to increase the amount of tissue harvested. This rationale could bypass the limitation of the ovarian reserve in some selected patients. Since age is closely related to follicular density and genetic quality of the gametes, in our program we do not perform ovarian cortex cryopreservation in patients over 35 years old unless they have AMH levels above 6 pM, and when done, the whole ovary is harvested.
3. Technical issues: If the amount of tissue is limited by the size of the ovary, for example, in pediatric patients, it could be preferable to harvest the whole ovary [65]. Despite all the abovementioned considerations, it has to be said that even doing a systematic oophorectomy/adnexectomy will not compromise significantly the ovarian reserve left after the oncologic treatment [66].

On the other hand, the reimplantation of just a few fragments of cortex has been proven to be effective with long lifespan and multiple pregnancies reported [64], and doing systematic oophorectomy will determine the technique used for reimplantation of the tissue (see Chap. 7).

4.3.2 Ovarian Tissue Transport and Manipulation

Any kind of tissue is sensitive to warm ischemia damage [67–71]. This is why ovarian tissue retrieval should be done close to the laboratory where the tissue is going to be processed in case the transport is going to be done at 37 °C or room temperature. Nevertheless, cold ischemia is much less detrimental for the tissue, and longer transport times can be done without compromising the viability of the ovary if temperatures are maintained between 4 and 10 °C. This is the case of centralized programs, like the Danish one, with transport times around 4–5 h being reported [62] and at least six live births after transplantation of the cryopreserved tissue [72]. In a similar multi-center setup in Germany, authors reported a case in which the tissue was transported during 20 h overnight [73]. The viability of the tissue was subsequently proven by a live birth [73].

The thickness of the ovarian fragments is one of the main causes of follicle survival because it determines the penetration rate of CPA during equilibration prior to cryopreservation and, on the other hand, the duration of the ischemia after transplantation. It has been described that only one-third of the transplanted follicles survives to the ischemia reperfusion damage [74]; thus, all the efforts to improve the efficiency of the technique should be focused on that issue. Then, the surface-to-volume ratio of the graft has to be high in order to ensure good penetration and evacuation of cryoprotective agents, to reduce the probability of damage caused by ice crystals during freezing and thawing, and to quickly overcome the ischemia and hypoxia that occur during the initial steps of graft reimplantation [75].

In human, primordial follicles can be found as deep as 0.8 mm from the tunica albuginea, but reducing too much the graft thickness in an attempt to improve freezing conditions can also have detrimental effects. Thinner biopsies can result in the absence of primordial follicles in the removed cortex [64] and in augmented follicular activation, which in the long term will reduce the lifespan of the graft [76]. Based on previous reports in the literature, most of them coming from experimental designs, we could conclude that a thickness between 0.75 and 1 mm could be optimal to allow for follicle cryoprotection as well as fast graft revascularization [59, 76–81], but they will show increased follicular activation when compared to fragments 1–2 mm thick [76, 77]. It is important to remark that in most of the programs, the ovarian cortical tissue is cryopreserved in strips of 1–2 mm [64].

Regarding the size of the transplanted ovarian grafts, there are several studies that proposed the use of squares, strips, and fragments ranging from 2–3 mm^2 to 1 cm^2 [82–85]. Nevertheless, to date, the best results have been achieved when bigger fragments were transplanted [64, 72, 86], obtaining ovarian function restoration with even only one fragment of ovarian tissue [87]. The explanation of such results could rely in the fact that tissue fragmentation can disrupt growth inhibition pathways (Salvador-Hippo route) resulting in increased primordial follicle activation [88] and follicular pool burnout.

4.3.3 Cryopreservation by Slow Freezing

The first attempt of ovarian cryopreservation was developed by Parkes in the 1950s to restore the endocrine function in ovariectomized rodents [89–93]. Glycerol was used as cryoprotectant, and the tissue was stored at −80 °C. Ovarian function was resumed after subcutaneous or orthotopic transplantation of those rudimentary cryopreserved ovarian grafts, and healthy offspring was also produced. Despite these encouraging results, there was no place yet to consider ovarian cryopreservation as a strategy. The surgical approaches and methods to cryopreserve the ovary that served as the base of FP in the human were mainly developed using the sheep [74, 78, 94] as an animal model. These later studies showed the seed of the future interest on ovarian tissue cryopreservation as a suitable technique for FP. The first experience developed with orthotopic transplantation of cryopreserved/thawed human ovarian tissue in cancer patients successfully restored the endocrine ovarian function of the patient already in 2001 [95]. The first proof of full restoration of ovarian activity took place in 2005 when Donnez's group reported for the first time a live birth after ovarian cortex slow-freezing cryopreservation and reimplantation [96]. Since then, more than 60 live births have been reported so far all around the world [97].

4.3.3.1 Cryoprotectants and Slow-Freezing Protocols

Successful cryopreservation requires the inclusion of molar concentrations of CPAs to the medium. The colligative properties of these agents induce the reduction of the freezing point and the probability of ice formation. This can be achieved by minimizing the growth of extracellular salt crystals and the intracellular ice formation [98]. Nevertheless, the toxicity induced by this compounds into cells requires that equilibration of CPA should be developed at low temperature during a short time and by using their lowest possible concentration. There is a fine line between cryoprotection and toxicity that should be taken into account when establishing the freezing procedure. A cryoprotectant is essential for survival after freezing and thawing, and the success of the cryopreservation procedure varied depending on the substance employed as a CPA. The choice of a suitable cryoprotectant solution is essential to ensure cell survival in ovarian tissue, being necessary a proper penetration of the CPA through stromal and granulosa cells, to the oocyte, avoiding at the same time any possible toxicity associated to high concentrations of CPA [99]. In general, the CPAs used to cryopreserve ovarian tissue are DMSO, glycerol (GLY), PROH, acetamide, formamide, and EG, being the last one the most commonly used, alone or in combination with other compounds [100–107].

One of the first reports to assess the effect of several CPAs in ovarian samples was developed by Newton [108] with human ovarian samples of 1 mm^3 of thickness that were cryoprotected with 1.5 M of EG, DMSO, PROH, or GLY during 30 min. They established that there were no significant differences between the results with EG, DMSO, and PROH, despite a large number of observations. Nevertheless, survival in GLY was poor [108]. A feasible explanation for that finding could be that GLY is more viscous than the other tested compounds; thus their penetration within the cells was inefficient leading to a lower protection against freezing injuries [98]. This study was just the first of a series that systematically tested the use of different compounds, concentrations, and exposure times to CPAs, and it established 30 min as the optimal time that balanced proper penetration within the tissue and harmless toxicity.

Further experiments tested the permeation rate of CPA agents for various periods of times at temperatures ranging from 0 to 37 °C [109–115]. They established that an incubation with 1.5 M DMSO or EG, during 15–30 min at 4 °C, is the most efficient equilibration procedure for human ovarian tissue cryopreservation [109, 115]. The perfect protocol for ovarian tissue slow freezing does not exist, and regardless of the CPA used or the exposure times, primordial follicular loss between 25 and 70 % has been described [111, 116–119].

To give the reader a broad view of the different protocols that can be applied, all the slow-freezing cryopreservation protocols used in clinical practice whose application has resulted in at least one pregnancy have been summarized in Table 4.1.

Table 4.1 Characteristics of the cryopreservation protocols used in the clinical setup and reporting at least one live birth

Author	Ovarian tissue	Equilibration freezing solution	Device	Cooling rate	Thawing	Cryoinjury
Silber et al. [63]	Tissue was divided into multiple strips	Equilibration in 1.5 M 1,2-PrOH 0.1 M sucrose at 37 for 30 min., followed by 1.5 M 1,2-PrOH and 0.2 M sucrose for 5 min	1.5 ml cryovials	2 °C/min to −7 °C, 0.3 °C/min to −30 °C, 50 ° C/min to −150 °C. Manual seed	Thawing was achieved rapidly by agitating 2–3 min the vials in a warmed water bath. Gradual dilution of cryoprotectant	Most of the stroma cells were lyzed and their nuclei compressed between dense bundles of extra-cellular fibers. Oocyte viability was less than one-half (42 %)
Demeestere et al. [34]	40 pieces (5 × 5 × 2 mm) of ovarian cortex.	Leibovitz medium supplemented with 1.5 M DMSO, 0.1 M sucrose, and 10 % patient's serum. Samples were equilibrated for 30 min. at 4 °C	2 ml vial, containing 1.4 ml of CPA solution	Planer freezer (Planner Kryo 360–3.3). The following program was used: started at 4 °C, 2 °C/min to –7 °C, 10 min of soaking, then manual seeding, 0.3 °C/min to –40 °C, 10 °C/min to –140 °C, and then plunged into liquid nitrogen	Vials were placed 2 min at RT and then 2 min in water at 25 °C. The ovarian tissue was washed stepwise for 5 min each in progressively lower concentrations of cryoprotectant solution (1.5, 1, 0.5, and 0 mol/l)	The follicles that developed at the subcutaneous site never reached sufficient size to be punctured at the time of ovulation (maximum 13 mm)
Roux et al. [126]	Eight ovarian cortical fragments (1 cm/0.5 cm).	Freezing solution containing 1.5 M DMSO and 0.1 M sucrose in Leibovitz L-15 medium supplemented with	Cryovials	Slow cooling with manual seeding	Quickly thawing the vials, the strips were washed in decreased solutions of DMSO 1.5 M (5 min.), 1 M	Viability of the tissue assessed by trypan blue staining of isolated follicles was 73 %, compared with 100 %

(continued)

Table 4.1 (continued)

Author	Ovarian tissue	Equilibration freezing solution	Device	Cooling rate	Thawing	Cryoinjury
		10 % decomplemented patient serum			(5 min.), 0.5 M (10 min.), and in a solution of 0.05 M sucrose in Leibovitz L-15 medium supplemented with 10 % decomplemented patient serum	before cryopreservation. Histology of the ovarian thawed strip revealed the presence of well-preserved follicles
Dittrich et al. [73]	Pieces measuring 1 × 2 × 1 mm	Freezing solution containing 1.5 M DMSO in Leibovitz medium with 0.1 M sucrose and 10 % synthetic substitute serum and were cooled in ice water (0–8 °C)	1.8 ml Nunc cryovials	1) The starting temperature was at 2 8C; 2) cooling from 2 8C to K6 8C at a rate of K2 8C/min; 3) auto-seeding initiated at K6 8C; 4) after beginning of crystal formation, the temperature increased to K5.7 8C and remained at this temperature for 10 min; 5) cooling from K5.7 8C to K40 8C at a rate of K0.3 8C/min; 6) cooling to K140 8C at a rate of K10 8C/min and plunging of cryovials into liquid nitrogen	Thawing was fast in a water bath with warm water (100 °C) during 60s. The tissue fragments were released from the CPA medium in reverse order with the addition of 0.25 M sucrose	

Revel et al. [127].	Ovarian cortex tissue was manually cut into slivers varying in size from 0.8 to 1.4 cm in length, 2–4 mm in depth, and 1.5–2.0 mm in width	Freezing solution containing 1.5 M DMSO in Leibovitz medium with 10 % serum	Cryovials	Cooled at 2 °C/min to −9 °C; (u) seeded manually; (iii) cooled at 0.3 °C/min to −40 °C; (iv) cooled to −140 °C at the higher rate of 10 °C/min; (v) plunged into liquid nitrogen	The vials were thawed individually by agitating in water at room temperature (~100 °C/min). The CPA was quickly removed from the tissue by repeated washing in saline and fresh Leibovitz medium	
Andersen et al. [128]	The cortex was isolated, cut into fragments of 5 × 5 mm (1–2 mm thickness)	After rinsed with isotonic saline solution, the pieces were transferred to 30 ml of 0.1 M sucrose and 1.5 M EG in PBS and equilibrated for 30 min at 1 °C on a tilting table	1.8 ml cryovials (Nunc A/S, Roskilde, Denmark), each containing 1 ml of cryoprotectant	Planer freezer (Planner K10). The following program was used: 2 °C/min to –9 °C, 5 min of soaking, then manual seeding for ice crystal nucleation induction, 0.3 °C/min to –40 °C, 10 °C/min to –140 °C, at which temperature the samples were plunged into liquid nitrogen at –196 °C	Samples were thawed rapidly in a 37 °C water bath	
Sanchez-Serrano et al. [87, 112]	In 95 % of cases, a piece (or two) of ovarian cortex sized ≥2 × 3 cm was obtained	The CPA solution contains 5 % of human serum albumin (HSA) and 12.5 % of DMSO in M199 culture medium. The addition of	Hemofreeze® Kapton-Teflon bags	Slow-freezing protocol with seven cooling ramps: (1) at 1 °C/min to −8 °C, (2) at 5 °C/min to −20 °C, (3) at 2.5 °C/min to −15 °C/min, (4) hold at −15 °C for 9 min, (5) at 0.5 °C/min to	Thawing was performed using an immersion bath at 42 °C. The CPA was gradually removed from the bag and replaced by M199 solution	

(continued)

Table 4.1 (continued)

Author	Ovarian tissue	Equilibration freezing solution	Device	Cooling rate	Thawing	Cryoinjury
		cryoprotectant was performed by sequential dilution in two steps		−35 °C, (6) at 5 °C/min to −60 °C, and (7) at 10 °C/min to −120 °C; 8 °C/min seeding was performed in step 2		
Rodriguez-Wallberg et al. [118, 129]	97 pieces of 1 × 3 × 5 mm	CPA solution was 1.5 M propanediol and 0.1 M sucrose in a-MEM supplemented with 20 % human serum at room temperature. Samples were incubated during 10 min and then submitted to SF	Vials (Nunc freezing vials; Nunclon, Roskilde, Denmark)	Programmable freezer, at a starting temperature of 18 °C, then was cooled at 2 °C/min to −8 °C. After being held at that temperature for 5 min, ice crystal formation was induced. After a further 10 min they were cooled at −0.3 °C/min to −30 °C and then at −50 °C/min to −150 °C	Vials were kept in air for 30 s and immersed in a water bath at 30 °C, then were transferred to 0.2 M sucrose in a-MEM containing decreasing concentrations of propanediol (1.0 M and 0.5 M) during 5 min, and finally were washed 10 min in medium with 0.2 M sucrose	There was no identifiable difference in histological examination before and after freezing. Follicles at varying developmental stages were found. Oocyte morphology was similar before and after freezing
Donnez et al. [64, 96]	70 small cubes of 2 × 2 mm, and one strip of 12 × 4 mm	Leibovitz medium supplemented with 4 mg/mL of human serum albumin and 1.5 M DMSO	2 mL cryogenic vials	Programmable freezer (Kryo 10, Series III; Planer) with the following program: (1) cooled from 0 °C to –8 °C at –2 °C/min; (2) seeded manually by touching the cryotubes with forceps	Tissue was thawed at room temperature (21 °C–23 °C) for 2 min and then immersed in a water bath at 37 °C for 2 min. Ovarian tissue was	Vital fluorescent staining confirmed survival of all primordial follicles after freeze thawing, while no primordial follicles were noted in serial

				prechilled in liquid nitrogen; (3) cooled to –40 °C at –0·3 °C/min; (4) cooled to –150 °C at –30 °C/min; and (5) transferred to liquid nitrogen (–196 °C) immediately for storage	immediately transferred from the vials to tissue culture dishes in Leibovitz medium and washed 3 times with fresh medium to remove cryoprotectant	sections of the biopsy taken from the atrophic ovaries. Follicular density was between 4 and 5 follicles per uL
Stern et al. [130, 131]	<1/4 of the ovary surface chopped in 4 × 2 mm strips	1.5 M propanediol with 0.1 M sucrose in base medium (10 mg/HSA in PBS) at room temperature for 90 min	2 ml cryogenic vials (Nunc A/S, Roskilde, Denmark), containing 1 ml of dehydration solution	Planer K10 automated freezing machine. The procedure started at room temperature, then was cooled at 2 °C/min to −8 °C, then manual seeded, and then cooled at −0.3 °C/min to −30 °C and then at −50 °C/min to −150 °C	Tissue was thawed in a water bath at 37 °C. Cryoprotectants were removed by a stepwise reduction of the PROH concentration with a final one-step dilution of the sucrose	Tested in a xenograft mouse model. The animals were followed up for 27 weeks, and 63 % presented antral follicles at examination

4.3.3.2 Cryopreservation Devices

Although the use of an adequate freezing solution is one of the main determinants of the cryopreservation technique success, the device employed to store the tissue has also a key role on the process. Several systems to cryopreserve ovarian tissue have been employed; this includes the widely used 1.8 ml cryovials, cryopreservation bags, metallic grids, electronic microscopy grids, and needles [59, 77, 120–123]. The use of the same freezing solution with diverse cryopreservation devices has been evaluated obtaining significant differences when the ovarian tissue preservation and follicular viability were assessed [111, 113, 123]. These findings indicate that the cryopreservation loading device plays a main role in cooling transmission inside the tissue and therefore could compromise the final outcome [123].

4.3.3.3 Limitations of Slow Freezing

The main problem associated to slow freezing, in spite of being the elective technique nowadays, is that it takes several hours and a programmable freezer is required to control the cooling rate. These limitations make impossible to perform the technique in many laboratories.

Regarding the efficiency to preserve the tissue, an increased induction of apoptotic processes after warming ovarian cortex cryopreserved by slow freezing [104, 111, 124] and also a decreased efficiency to preserve all types of ovarian cells, especially in the ovarian cortex stroma [117] and granulosa cells [122], when compared with the new vitrification techniques have also been noted. Furthermore, after slow freezing, the preservation of follicles and the ovarian stroma was very variable. The obtained values for follicular survival ranged from 28 %[117] to 91 % [116] in primordial follicles, depending on the employed CPA, and from 42 %[119] to 73 %[118] when the primary follicle population was analyzed. In all cases, although survival of stromal cells reached high values [116], an inefficient preservation of vessels in the ovarian stroma was described [99, 116–119]. It has been shown that vitrification could help to preserve the stroma and the vessels better than slow freezing [111, 122], but it has to be highlighted that the only valid endpoint is live birth and the current clinical experience in the field of FP is limited to slow freezing [72], although at least two live births after vitrification of ovarian tissue have been reported in premature ovarian failure patients [125]. To date, it seems reasonable to move to vitrification only in the setup of clinical trials.

References

1. Linabery AM, Ross JA (2008) Childhood and adolescent cancer survival in the US by race and ethnicity for the diagnostic period 1975–1999. Cancer 113(9):2575–2596
2. Gnerlich JL, Deshpande AD, Jeffe DB, Sweet A, White N, Margenthaler JA (2009) Elevated breast cancer mortality in women younger than age 40 years compared with older women is attributed to poorer survival in early-stage disease. J Am Coll Surg 208(3):341–347
3. Jemal A, Clegg LX, Ward E, Ries LA, Wu X, Jamison PM et al (2004) Annual report to the nation on the status of cancer, 1975–2001, with a special feature regarding survival. Cancer 101(1):3–27
4. Marhhom E, Cohen I (2007) Fertility preservation options for women with malignancies. Obstet Gynecol Surv 62(1):58–72
5. Bleyer WA (1990) The impact of childhood cancer on the United States and the world. CA Cancer J Clin 40(6):355–367
6. Meirow D, Dor J, Kaufman B, Shrim A, Rabinovici J, Schiff E et al (2007) Cortical fibrosis and blood-vessels damage in human ovaries exposed to chemotherapy. Potential mechanisms of ovarian injury. Hum Reprod 22(6):1626–1633
7. Kiserud CE, Fossa A, Holte H, Fossa SD (2007) Post-treatment parenthood in Hodgkin's lymphoma survivors. Br J Cancer 96(9):1442–1449
8. Familiari G, Caggiati A, Nottola SA, Ermini M, Di Benedetto MR, Motta PM (1993) Ultrastructure of human ovarian primordial follicles after combination chemotherapy for Hodgkin's disease. Hum Reprod 8(12):2080–2087
9. Kalich-Philosoph L, Roness H, Carmely A, Fishel-Bartal M, Ligumsky H, Paglin S et al (2013) Cyclophosphamide triggers follicle activation and "burnout"; AS101 prevents follicle loss and preserves fertility. Sci Transl Med [Research Support, Non-US Gov't] 5 (185):185ra62
10. Meirow D, Baum M, Yaron R, Levron J, Hardan I, Schiff E et al (2007) Ovarian tissue cryopreservation in hematologic malignancy: ten years' experience. Leuk Lymphoma 48 (8):1569–1576
11. Chiarelli AM, Marrett LD, Darlington G (1999) Early menopause and infertility in females after treatment for childhood cancer diagnosed in 1964–1988 in Ontario Canada. Am J Epidemiol 150(3):245–254
12. Wallace WH, Thomson AB, Kelsey TW (2003) The radiosensitivity of the human oocyte. Hum Reprod 18(1):117–121
13. Grigsby PW, Herzog TJ (2001) Current management of patients with invasive cervical carcinoma. Clin Obstet Gynecol 44(3):531–537
14. Gill S, Blackstock AW, Goldberg RM (2007) Colorectal cancer. Mayo Clin Proc 82 (1):114–129
15. Tauchmanova L, Selleri C, Rosa GD, Pagano L, Orio F, Lombardi G et al (2002) High prevalence of endocrine dysfunction in long-term survivors after allogeneic bone marrow transplantation for hematologic diseases. Cancer 95(5):1076–1084
16. Linch DC, Gosden RG, Tulandi T, Tan SL, Hancock SL (2000) Hodgkin's lymphoma: choice of therapy and late complications. Hematol Am Soc Hematol Educ Program 205–221
17. Burdach S, van Kaick B, Laws HJ, Ahrens S, Haase R, Korholz D et al (2000) Allogeneic and autologous stem-cell transplantation in advanced Ewing tumors. An update after long-term follow-up from two centers of the European Intergroup study EICESS. Stem-Cell Transplant Programs at Dusseldorf University Medical Center, Germany and St. Anna Kinderspital, Vienna, Austria. Ann Oncol 11(11):1451–1462
18. Wu HY, Snyder HM 3rd, D'Angio GJ (2005) Wilms' tumor management. Curr Opin Urol 15 (4):273–276
19. Spreafico F, Bellani FF (2006) Wilms' tumor: past, present and (possibly) future. Expert Rev Anticancer Ther 6(2):249–258

20. Demeestere I, Simon P, Emiliani S, Delbaere A, Englert Y (2009) Orthotopic and heterotopic ovarian tissue transplantation. Hum Reprod Update [Research Support, Non-US Gov't Review] 15(6):649–665
21. Practice Committee of American Society for Reproductive M (2013) Fertility preservation in patients undergoing gonadotoxic therapy or gonadectomy: a committee opinion. Fertil Steril [Practice Guideline] 100(5):1214–1223
22. von Wolff M, Thaler CJ, Frambach T, Zeeb C, Lawrenz B, Popovici RM et al. (2009) Ovarian stimulation to cryopreserve fertilized oocytes in cancer patients can be started in the luteal phase. Fertil Steril 92(4):1360–1365
23. Maman E, Meirow D, Brengauz M, Raanani H, Dor J, Hourvitz A (2011) Luteal phase oocyte retrieval and in vitro maturation is an optional procedure for urgent fertility preservation. Fertil Steril 95(1):64–67
24. Fadini R, Mignini Renzini M, Dal Canto M, Epis A, Crippa M, Caliari I et al (2013) Oocyte in vitro maturation in normo-ovulatory women. Fertil Steril [Review] 99(5):1162–1169
25. Shaw JM, Jones GM (2003) Terminology associated with vitrification and other cryopreservation procedures for oocytes and embryos. Hum Reprod Update 9(6):583–605
26. Kuwayama M (2007) Highly efficient vitrification for cryopreservation of human oocytes and embryos: the Cryotop method. Theriogenology 67(1):73–80
27. Mazur P (1970) Cryobiology: the freezing of biological systems. Science 168(3934):939–949
28. Sun WQ (1999) State and phase transition behaviors of Quercus rubra seed axes and cotyledonary tissues: relevance to the desiccation sensitivity and cryopreservation of recalcitrant seeds. Cryobiology 38(4):372–385
29. Liebermann J (2002) Potential importance of vitrification in reproductive medicine. Biol Reprod 67(6):1671–1680
30. Muldrew K, McGann LE (1990) Mechanisms of intracellular ice formation. Biophys J 57 (3):525–532
31. Mazur P (1990) Equilibrium, quasi-equilibrium, and nonequilibrium freezing of mammalian embryos. Cell Biophys 17(1):53–92
32. Shaw JM, Oranratnachai A, Trounson AO (2000) Fundamental cryobiology of mammalian oocytes and ovarian tissue. Theriogenology 53(1):59–72
33. Whittingham DG, Leibo SP, Mazur P (1972) Survival of mouse embryos frozen to −196 and −269 C. Science 178(4059):411–414
34. Demeestere I, Simon P, Buxant F, Robin V, Fernandez SA, Centner J et al (2006) Ovarian function and spontaneous pregnancy after combined heterotopic and orthotopic cryopreserved ovarian tissue transplantation in a patient previously treated with bone marrow transplantation: case report. Hum Reprod 21(8):2010–2014
35. Shaw JM, Kola I, MacFarlane DR, Trounson AO (1991) An association between chromosomal abnormalities in rapidly frozen 2-cell mouse embryos and the ice-forming properties of the cryoprotective solution. Reproduction 91(1):9–18
36. Arav A, Natan Y (2009) Directional freezing: a solution to the methodological challenges to preserve large organs. Semin Reprod Med 27(06):438–442
37. Wowk B (2010) Thermodynamic aspects of vitrification. Cryobiology 60(1):11–22
38. Fahy GM (2010) Cryoprotectant toxicity neutralization. Cryobiology 60(3):S45–S53
39. Karlsson JOM, Toner M (1996) Long-term storage of tissues by cryopreservation: critical issues. Biomaterials 17(3):243–256
40. Acker JP, Elliott JAW, McGann LE (2001) Intercellular ice propagation: experimental evidence for ice growth through membrane pores. Biophys J 81(3):1389–1397
41. Beckmann J, Körber C, Rau G, Hubel A, Cravalho EG (1990) Redefining cooling rate in terms of ice front velocity and thermal gradient: first evidence of relevance to freezing injury of lymphocytes. Cryobiology 27(3):279–287
42. Hubel A, Cravalho EG, Nunner B, Körber C (1992) Survival of directionally solidified B-lymphoblasts under various crystal growth conditions. Cryobiology 29(2):183–198

43. Rall WF, Reid DS, Polge C (1984) Analysis of slow-warming injury of mouse embryos by cryomicroscopical and physiochemical methods. Cryobiology 21(1):106–121
44. Gougeon A (1996) Regulation of ovarian follicular development in primates: facts and hypotheses. Endocr Rev 17(2):121–155
45. Qu J, Godin PA, Nisolle M, Donnez J (2000) Distribution and epidermal growth factor receptor expression of primordial follicles in human ovarian tissue before and after cryopreservation. Hum Reprod 15(2):302–310
46. Picton HM, Harris SE, Muruvi W, Chambers EL (2008) The in vitro growth and maturation of follicles. Reproduction 136(6):703–715
47. Thomas FH, Walters KA, Telfer EE (2003) How to make a good oocyte: an update on in-vitro models to study follicle regulation. Hum Reprod Update 9(6):541–555
48. Zuckerman S (1951) The number of oocytes in the mature ovary. Recent Prog Horm Res 6:63–108
49. Tingen CM, Bristol-Gould SK, Kiesewetter SE, Wellington JT, Shea L, Woodruff TK (2009) Prepubertal primordial follicle loss in mice is not due to classical apoptotic pathways. Biol Reprod 81(1):16–25
50. Hardy K, Wright CS, Franks S, Winston RM (2000) In vitro maturation of oocytes. Br Med Bull 56(3):588–602
51. Hansen KR, Knowlton NS, Thyer AC, Charleston JS, Soules MR, Klein NA (2008) A new model of reproductive aging: the decline in ovarian non-growing follicle number from birth to menopause. Hum Reprod 23(3):699–708
52. Macklon NS, Fauser BC (1999) Aspects of ovarian follicle development throughout life. Horm Res 52(4):161–170
53. Greenwald GS (1972) Of eggs and follicles. Am J Anat 135(1):1–3
54. Lass A (2004) Assessment of ovarian reserve: is there still a role for ovarian biopsy in the light of new data? Hum Reprod [Review] 19(3):467–469
55. Kohl J, Dittrich R, Siebzehnrübl E, Wildt L (2000) Determination of follicle numbers in human ovarian biopsies—a method for estimation of outcome of ovarian cryopreservation? Fertil Steril 74(3):1
56. Poirot C, Vacher-Lavenu MC, Helardot P, Guibert J, Brugieres L, Jouannet P (2002) Human ovarian tissue cryopreservation: indications and feasibility. Hum Reprod 17(6):1447–1452
57. Schmidt KL, Byskov AG, Nyboe Andersen A, Muller J, Yding Andersen C (2003) Density and distribution of primordial follicles in single pieces of cortex from 21 patients and in individual pieces of cortex from three entire human ovaries. Hum Reprod 18(6):1158–1164
58. Kristensen SG, Rasmussen A, Byskov AG, Andersen CY (2011) Isolation of pre-antral follicles from human ovarian medulla tissue. Hum Reprod [Research Support, Non-US Gov't] 26(1):157–166
59. Kagawa N, Kuwayama M, Nakata K, Vajta G, Silber S, Manabe N et al (2007) Production of the first offspring from oocytes derived from fresh and cryopreserved pre-antral follicles of adult mice. Reprod Biomed Online 14(6):693–699
60. Shimizu T, Jiang JY, Iijima K, Miyabayashi K, Ogawa Y, Sasada H et al (2003) Induction of follicular development by direct single injection of vascular endothelial growth factor gene fragments into the ovary of miniature gilts. Biol Reprod 69(4):1388–1393
61. Nunez Valera MJ, Padilla Iserte P, Higueras Garcia G, Herraiz S, Rubio JM, Romeu Villarroya M et al (2015) Single site laparoscopy for fertility preservation: a cohort study. J Minim Invasive Gynecol 22(2):291–296
62. Rosendahl M, Schmidt KT, Ernst E, Rasmussen PE, Loft A, Byskov AG et al (2011) Cryopreservation of ovarian tissue for a decade in Denmark: a view of the technique. Reprod Biomed Online [Historical Article Research Support, Non-US Gov't] 22(2):162–171
63. Silber S, Kagawa N, Kuwayama M, Gosden R (2010) Duration of fertility after fresh and frozen ovary transplantation. Fertil Steril 94(6):2191–2196
64. Donnez J, Dolmans MM, Pellicer A, Diaz-Garcia C, Sanchez Serrano M, Schmidt KT et al (2013) Restoration of ovarian activity and pregnancy after transplantation of

cryopreserved ovarian tissue: a review of 60 cases of reimplantation. Fertil Steril 99 (6):1503–1513
65. Jadoul P, Dolmans MM, Donnez J (2010) Fertility preservation in girls during childhood: is it feasible, efficient and safe and to whom should it be proposed? Hum Reprod Update [Research Support, Non-US Gov't Review] 16(6):617–630
66. Rosendahl M, Andersen CY, Ernst E, Westergaard LG, Rasmussen PE, Loft A et al (2008) Ovarian function after removal of an entire ovary for cryopreservation of pieces of cortex prior to gonadotoxic treatment: a follow-up study. Hum Reprod 23(11):2475–2483
67. Cursio R, Colosetti P (2015) Autophagy and liver ischemia-reperfusion injury. Biomed Res Int 2015:417590
68. Gonzalez LM, Moeser AJ, Blikslager AT (2015) Animal models of ischemia-reperfusion-induced intestinal injury: progress and promise for translational research. Am J Physiol Gastrointest Liver Physiol 308(2):G63–G75
69. Hilbert T, Klaschik S (2015) The angiopoietin/TIE receptor system: focusing its role for ischemia-reperfusion injury. Cytokine Growth Factor Rev 26(3):281–291
70. Ibanez B, Heusch G, Ovize M, Van de Werf F (2015) Evolving therapies for myocardial ischemia/reperfusion injury. BioMed Res Int 65(14):1454–1471
71. Salvadori M, Rosso G, Bertoni E (2015) Update on ischemia-reperfusion injury in kidney transplantation: pathogenesis and treatment. World J Trans 5(2):52–67
72. Donnez J, Dolmans MM, Pellicer A, Diaz-Garcia C, Ernst E, Macklon KT et al (2015) Fertility preservation for age-related fertility decline. Lancet [Comment Letter] 385 (9967):506–507
73. Dittrich R, Lotz L, Keck G, Hoffmann I, Mueller A, Beckmann MW et al (2012) Live birth after ovarian tissue autotransplantation following overnight transportation before cryopreservation. Fertil Steril 97(2):387–390
74. Baird DT, Webb R, Campbell BK, Harkness LM, Gosden RG (1999) Long-term ovarian function in sheep after ovariectomy and transplantation of autografts stored at -196 C. Endocrinology 140(1):462–471
75. Gavish Z, Ben-Haim M, Arav A (2008) Cryopreservation of whole murine and porcine livers. Rejuvenation Res 11(4):765–772
76. Gavish Z, Peer G, Roness H, Cohen Y, Meirow D (2014) Follicle activation and 'burn-out' contribute to post-transplantation follicle loss in ovarian tissue grafts: the effect of graft thickness. Hum Reprod [Research Support, Non-US Gov't] 29(5):989–996
77. Kagawa N, Silber S, Kuwayama M (2009) Successful vitrification of bovine and human ovarian tissue. Reprod Biomed Online 18(4):568–577
78. Gosden RG, Baird DT, Wade JC, Webb R (1994) Restoration of fertility to oophorectomized sheep by ovarian autografts stored at -196 degrees C. Hum Reprod 9(4):597–603
79. Silber SJ, DeRosa M, Pineda J, Lenahan K, Grenia D, Gorman K et al (2008) A series of monozygotic twins discordant for ovarian failure: ovary transplantation (cortical versus microvascular) and cryopreservation. Hum Reprod 23(7):1531–1537
80. Arav A, Zeron Y, Leslie SB, Behboodi E, Anderson GB, Crowe JH (1996) Phase transition temperature and chilling sensitivity of bovine oocytes. Cryobiology 33(6):589–599
81. Silber SJ, Grudzinskas G, Gosden RG (2008) Successful pregnancy after microsurgical transplantation of an intact ovary. N Engl J Med 359(24):2617–2618
82. Oktay K, Karlikaya G (2000) Ovarian function after transplantation of frozen, banked autologous ovarian tissue. N Engl J Med 342(25):1919
83. Callejo J, Salvador C, Miralles A, Vilaseca S, Lailla JM, Balasch J (2001) Long-term ovarian function evaluation after autografting by implantation with fresh and frozen-thawed human ovarian tissue. J Clin Endocrinol Metab 86(9):4489–4494
84. Gook DA, McCully BA, Edgar DH, McBain JC (2001) Development of antral follicles in human cryopreserved ovarian tissue following xenografting. Hum Reprod 16(3):417–422

85. Oktay K, Buyuk E, Veeck L, Zaninovic N, Xu K, Takeuchi T et al (2004) Embryo development after heterotopic transplantation of cryopreserved ovarian tissue. Lancet 363 (9412):837–840
86. Meirow D, Levron J, Eldar-Geva T, Hardan I, Fridman E, Zalel Y et al (2005) Pregnancy after transplantation of cryopreserved ovarian tissue in a patient with ovarian failure after chemotherapy. N Engl J Med 353(3):318–321
87. Sanchez-Serrano M, Crespo J, Mirabet V, Cobo AC, Escriba MJ, Simon C et al (2010) Twins born after transplantation of ovarian cortical tissue and oocyte vitrification. Fertil Steril 93 (1):268 e11–3
88. Kawamura K, Cheng Y, Suzuki N, Deguchi M, Sato Y, Takae S et al (2013) Hippo signaling disruption and Akt stimulation of ovarian follicles for infertility treatment. Proc Natl Acad Sci U S A 110(43):17474–17479
89. Parkes AS (1953) Conservation of gonadal tissue for transplantation. Acta Physiol Lat Am 3 (2–3):158–161
90. Parkes AS (1956) Grafting of mouse ovarian tissue after freezing and thawing. J Endocrinol 14(3):xxx--xxxi
91. Parkes AS (1956) Survival time of ovarian homografts in two strains of rats. J Endocrinol 13 (2):201–210
92. Parkes AS (1957) Viability of ovarian tissue after freezing. Proc R Soc Lond Ser B Biol Sci 147(929):520–528
93. Parkes AS, Smith AU (1953) Regeneration of rat ovarian tissue grafted after exposure to low temperatures. Proc R Soc Lond Ser B Biol Sci 140(901):455–470
94. Baird DT, Campbell B, de Souza C, Telfer E (2004) Long-term ovarian function in sheep after ovariectomy and autotransplantation of cryopreserved cortical strips. Eur J Obstet Gynecol Reprod Biol 113(Suppl 1):S55–S59
95. Radford JA, Lieberman BA, Brison DR, Smith AR, Critchlow JD, Russell SA et al (2001) Orthotopic reimplantation of cryopreserved ovarian cortical strips after high-dose chemotherapy for Hodgkin's lymphoma. Lancet 357(9263):1172–1175
96. Donnez J, Dolmans MM, Demylle D, Jadoul P, Pirard C, Squifflet J et al (2004) Livebirth after orthotopic transplantation of cryopreserved ovarian tissue. Lancet 364 (9443):1405–1410
97. Donnez J, Dolmans MM (2015) Ovarian cortex transplantation: 60 reported live births brings the success and worldwide expansion of the technique towards routine clinical practice. J Assist Reprod Genet 32:1167–1170. doi:10.1007/s10815-015-0544-9
98. Ashwood-Smith MJ (1986) The cryopreservation of human embryos. Hum Reprod 1 (5):319–332
99. Hovatta O (2005) Methods for cryopreservation of human ovarian tissue. Reprod Biomed Online 10(6):729–734
100. Gandolfi F, Paffoni A, Papasso Brambilla E, Bonetti S, Brevini TA, Ragni G (2006) Efficiency of equilibrium cooling and vitrification procedures for the cryopreservation of ovarian tissue: comparative analysis between human and animal models. Fertil Steril 85 (Suppl 1):1150–1156
101. Huang L, Mo Y, Wang W, Li Y, Zhang Q, Yang D (2008) Cryopreservation of human ovarian tissue by solid-surface vitrification. Eur J Obstet Gynecol Reprod Biol 139 (2):193–198
102. Isachenko V, Isachenko E, Rahimi G, Krivokharchenko A, Alabart JL, Nawroth F (2002) Cryopreservation of human ovarian tissue by direct plunging into liquid nitrogen: negative effect of disaccharides in vitrification solution. Cryo Lett 23(5):333–344
103. Isachenko E, Isachenko V, Rahimi G, Nawroth F (2003) Cryopreservation of human ovarian tissue by direct plunging into liquid nitrogen. Eur J Obstet Gynecol Reprod Biol 108 (2):186–193

104. Rahimi G, Isachenko E, Sauer H, Isachenko V, Wartenberg M, Hescheler J et al (2003) Effect of different vitrification protocols for human ovarian tissue on reactive oxygen species and apoptosis. Reprod Fertil Dev 15(6):343–349
105. Isachenko V, Isachenko E, Reinsberg J, Montag M, van der Ven K, Dorn C et al (2007) Cryopreservation of human ovarian tissue: comparison of rapid and conventional freezing. Cryobiology 55(3):261–268
106. Isachenko V, Isachenko E, Reinsberg J, Montag M, Weiss J, Braun F et al (2008) Simplified technique of human ovarian tissue freezing: quick cooling from -36 degree C. Cryo Lett 29 (3):261–268
107. Isachenko V, Isachenko E, Reinsberg J, Montag M, Braun F, van der Ven H (2008) Cryopreservation of human ovarian tissue: effect of spontaneous and initiated ice formation. Reprod Biomed Online 16(3):336–345
108. Newton H, Aubard Y, Rutherford A, Sharma V, Gosden R (1996) Low temperature storage and grafting of human ovarian tissue. Hum Reprod 11(7):1487–1491
109. Newton H, Fisher J, Arnold JR, Pegg DE, Faddy MJ, Gosden RG (1998) Permeation of human ovarian tissue with cryoprotective agents in preparation for cryopreservation. Hum Reprod 13(2):376–380
110. Candy CJ, Wood MJ, Whittingham DG (1997) Effect of cryoprotectants on the survival of follicles in frozen mouse ovaries. J Reprod Fertil 110(1):11–19
111. Herraiz S, Novella-Maestre E, Rodriguez B, Diaz C, Sanchez-Serrano M, Mirabet V et al (2014) Improving ovarian tissue cryopreservation for oncologic patients: slow freezing versus vitrification, effect of different procedures and devices. Fertil Steril 101(3):775–784
112. Sanchez M, Novella-Maestre E, Teruel J, Ortiz E, Pellicer A (2008) The Valencia Programme for fertility preservation. Clin Trans Oncol: Off Publ Fed Span Oncol Soc Natl Cancer Inst Mex 10(7):433–438
113. Amorim CA, David A, Van Langendonckt A, Dolmans MM, Donnez J (2011) Vitrification of human ovarian tissue: effect of different solutions and procedures. Fertil Steril 95 (3):1094–1097
114. Fahy GM, Wowk B, Wu J, Paynter S (2004) Improved vitrification solutions based on the predictability of vitrification solution toxicity. Cryobiology 48(1):22–35
115. Gook DA, Edgar DH, Stern C (2004) Cryopreservation of human ovarian tissue. Eur J Obstet Gynecol Reprod Biol 113(Suppl 1):S41–S44
116. Gook DA, Edgar DH, Stern C (2000) The effects of cryopreservation regimens on the morphology of human ovarian tissue. Mol Cell Endocrinol 169(1–2):99–103
117. Keros V, Xella S, Hultenby K, Pettersson K, Sheikhi M, Volpe A et al (2009) Vitrification versus controlled-rate freezing in cryopreservation of human ovarian tissue. Hum Reprod 24 (7):1670–1683
118. Hovatta O, Silye R, Krausz T, Abir R, Margara R, Trew G et al (1996) Cryopreservation of human ovarian tissue using dimethylsulphoxide and propanediol-sucrose as cryoprotectants. Hum Reprod 11(6):1268–1272
119. Maltaris T, Koelbl H, Fischl F, Seufert R, Schmidt M, Kohl J et al (2006) Xenotransplantation of human ovarian tissue pieces in gonadotropin-stimulated SCID mice: the effect of ovariectomy. Anticancer Res 26(6B):4171–4176
120. Chen SU, Chien CL, Wu MY, Chen TH, Lai SM, Lin CW et al (2006) Novel direct cover vitrification for cryopreservation of ovarian tissues increases follicle viability and pregnancy capability in mice. Hum Reprod 21(11):2794–2800
121. Oktem O, Alper E, Balaban B, Palaoglu E, Peker K, Karakaya C et al (2011) Vitrified human ovaries have fewer primordial follicles and produce less antimullerian hormone than slow-frozen ovaries. Fertil Steril 95(8):2661–2664, e1
122. Sheikhi M, Hultenby K, Niklasson B, Lundqvist M, Hovatta O (2011) Clinical grade vitrification of human ovarian tissue: an ultrastructural analysis of follicles and stroma in vitrified tissue. Hum Reprod 26(3):594–603

123. Zhou XH, Wu YJ, Shi J, Xia YX, Zheng SS (2010) Cryopreservation of human ovarian tissue: comparison of novel direct cover vitrification and conventional vitrification. Cryobiology 60(2):101–105
124. Mazoochi T, Salehnia M, Valojerdi MR, Mowla SJ (2008) Morphologic, ultrastructural, and biochemical identification of apoptosis in vitrified-warmed mouse ovarian tissue. Fertil Steril 90(4 Suppl):1480–1486
125. Suzuki N, Yoshioka N, Takae S, Sugishita Y, Tamura M, Hashimoto S et al (2015) Successful fertility preservation following ovarian tissue vitrification in patients with primary ovarian insufficiency. Hum Reprod [Research Support, Non-US Gov't] 30(3):608–615
126. Roux C, Amiot C, Agnani G, Aubard Y, Rohrlich PS, Piver P (2010) Live birth after ovarian tissue autograft in a patient with sickle cell disease treated by allogeneic bone marrow transplantation. Fertil Steril 93(7):2413, e15–9
127. Revel A, Laufer N, Ben Meir A, Lebovich M, Mitrani E (2011) Micro-organ ovarian transplantation enables pregnancy: a case report. Hum Reprod 26(5):1097–1103
128. Andersen CY, Rosendahl M, Byskov AG, Loft A, Ottosen C, Dueholm M et al (2008) Two successful pregnancies following autotransplantation of frozen/thawed ovarian tissue. Hum Reprod 23(10):2266–2272
129. Rodriguez-Wallberg KA, Karlstrom PO, Rezapour M, Castellanos E, Hreinsson J, Rasmussen C et al (2015) Full-term newborn after repeated ovarian tissue transplants in a patient treated for Ewing sarcoma by sterilizing pelvic irradiation and chemotherapy. Acta Obstet Gynecol Scand [Case Reports Research Support, Non-US Gov't] 94(3):324–328
130. Gook DA, Edgar DH, Stern C (1999) Effect of cooling rate and dehydration regimen on the histological appearance of human ovarian cortex following cryopreservation in 1, 2-propanediol. Hum Reprod 14(8):2061–2068
131. Stern CJ, Gook D, Hale LG, Agresta F, Oldham J, Rozen G et al (2014) Delivery of twins following heterotopic grafting of frozen-thawed ovarian tissue. Hum Reprod [Comment Letter] 29(8):1828

Chapter 5
Ovarian Tissue Cryopreservation: Ovarian Cortical Tissue Vitrification

Yodo Sugishita, Shu Hashimoto, Takayuki Yamochi, Suguru Igarashi, Mariko Nakajima, Chie Nishijima, Seido Takae, Yuki Horage, Kazuhiro Kawaura, Yoshihiko Hosoi, Yoshiharu Morimoto, and Nao Suzuki

Abstract Vitrification has become common practice in cryopreservation of embryo, blastocyst, oocytes, and sperm. Freezing of ovarian tissue has been studied since the late 1990s, and in 2004, Donnez et al. reported that live births could be achieved with this method. Reports worldwide have indicated that slow freezing is a common method of cryopreservation. Successive reports have emerged since 2005 describing ovarian tissue cryopreservation by vitrification in animal experiments and using human tissue; however, there have been no reports to date in which vitrification was clinically applied and live births were successfully achieved. We have been conducting studies through pre-clinical tests using Cynomolgus monkey (*Macaca fascicularis*) since 2006, and as a result, at present in June, 2016, we have achieved ovarian tissue cryopreservation in 229 cases and 2 live births following thawed transplantation. This article outlines the research findings so far regarding ovarian tissue cryopreservation by vitrification; additionally, it describes our ovarian cortical tissue vitrification method.

Keywords Fertility preservation • Slow freezing • Vitrification • Ovarian tissue cryopreservation • Ovarian cortical tissue vitrification • Ovarian cortex vitrifycation

---

Y. Sugishita • S. Igarashi • M. Nakajima • C. Nishijima • S. Takae • Y. Horage • K. Kawaura • N. Suzuki (✉)
Department of Obstetrics and Gynecology, St. Marianna University School of Medicine, 2-16-1 Sugao, Miyamae-ku, Kawasaki, Kanagawa 216-8511, Japan
e-mail: nao@marianna-u.ac.jp

S. Hashimoto • T. Yamochi
IVF Namba Clinic, Osaka, Japan

Y. Hosoi
Institute of Advanced Technology, Kinki University, Wakayama, Japan

Y. Morimoto
IVF Namba Clinic, Osaka, Japan

Horac Grand Front Osaka Clinic, Osaka, Japan

N. Suzuki, J. Donnez (eds.), *Gonadal Tissue Cryopreservation in Fertility Preservation*, DOI 10.1007/978-4-431-55963-4_5

5.1 Background

Vitrification (ultra-rapid freezing method) is widely considered to be a technique mostly performed to freeze embryos, blastocysts, sperms, and oocytes. On searching "vitrification" in the PubMed database, we found 2840 relevant publications, of which the oldest report was published by Hoagland et al. in 1942, titled "Revival of mammalian sperm after immersion in liquid nitrogen" [1].

Remarkable scientific advancements in recent years have enabled the long-term preservation of blood and cells in liquid nitrogen. With this technology, cryopreservation is being established for female reproductive cells, including embryos, blastocysts, and oocytes. Furthermore, despite the increasing prevalence of cancer among young adults with the accuracy of diagnosis increasing with medical advancements, the survival rates are increasing because of a wider array of available treatment options. However, in such patients, although the administration of anticancer agents and radiation therapy improves survival, fertility may be reduced or lost. With an aim to improve the quality of life (QOL) of young cancer patients following anticancer treatment, fertility-preserving treatment to cryopreserve reproductive cells before initiation of anticancer treatment, has been started already.

The American Society of Reproductive Medicine (ASRM) currently recognizes ovarian tissue cryopreservation is an option to preserve reproductive potential in patients who must urgently undergo aggressive chemotherapy and/or radiotherapy or who have other medical conditions requiring treatment that may threaten ovarian function and subsequent fertility. Ovarian tissue cryopreservation may be the only option available to prepubertal girls undergoing such treatments. However, these techniques are still considered to be experimental [2]. At present, ovarian tissue cryopreservation is considered an established technique in Europe, and ovarian tissue cryopreservation has drawn attention for various other reasons.

For many patients, upon detection of cancer, treatment proceeds rapidly with surgery, chemotherapy, and radiation therapy, leaving no scope for the patient and the attending physician to take into consideration the fertility issue prior to such treatments. As the start of anticancer treatment approaches, there is no scope for time extension, and despite fertility-related concerns following anticancer treatment, it is extremely difficult to preserve fertility without postponing anticancer treatment. Regarding preservation of fertility using oocytes, embryos, and lastocyst, oocytes are harvested depending on the menstrual cycle, thereby making it extremely difficult to harvest, in a short period, the number of oocytes required to actually conceive. In other words, fertility preserving treatment becomes inadequate. In 2013, a stimulation method called the random-start controlled ovarian stimulation that is independent of the menstrual cycle was reported [3]. However, in the event that only few days are available, it is extremely difficult to harvest eggs and preserve fertility even with this method. On the other hand, fertility-preserving treatment involving unilateral ovary removal by laparoscopic surgery and subsequent ovarian tissue cryopreservation only requires a single day and can be performed even when not much time is available. If the original ovarian function can be achieved following cryopreserved-thawed transplantation, ova can be permanently preserved in a short period without depending on the menstrual cycle in numbers higher than required for in-vitro fertilization, although the ovarian function depends on age.

Ovarian tissue cryopreservation has been examined since before 2000 [4–9], and in 2004, Oktay et al. reported that embryos could be harvested from ovarian tissue following freeze-thawed transplantation [10]. Thereafter Donnez et al. reported that with this method, conception can occur [11], and thus, ovarian tissue freezing techniques were fully implemented and explored further.

5.2 Various Guidelines for Ovarian Tissue Cryopreservation

In general fertility treatments, freezing technology has shown an improving progress from slow freezing to vitrification (ultra-rapid freezing). This flow is the same for fertility-preserving methods for young cancer patients excluding ovarian tissue freezing. Regarding ovarian tissue, 12 years have passed since Donnez et al. reported successful live births in 2004; however, slow freezing is the standard cryopreservation method adopted worldwide, and various reports of ovarian tissue cryopreservation have been published [12–22]. Based on a report from Stoop et al. [23], Donnez et al. (2015) reported the fertility rate of frozen ovarian tissue [24], according to Donnez et al.'s the fertility rate following the transplantation of freeze-thawed ovarian tissue is 25 %. In 2011, the guidelines on ovarian tissue freezing were first published by the FertiPROTEKT network with respect to ovarian tissue cryopreservation [25]. The guidelines recommended that ovarian tissue cryopreservation could be indicated for patients with breast cancer, Hodgkin's disease, and borderline ovarian tumors (ovarian borderline malignant tumors). Soon after, in 2012, the International Society for Fertility Preservation (ISFP) reported ovarian tissue cryopreservation guidelines for patients with lymphoma, leukemia, and breast cancer [26]. In 2013, the American Society of Clinical Oncology (ASCO) renewed their guidelines titled "Fertility Preservation for Patients with Cancer" [27]; however, the new ASCO guideline did not take into account the different malignancies, and ovarian tissue cryopreservation was considered an experimental procedure and was not specifically mentioned therein. In 2014, the Adolescent and Young Adult Oncology, version 2.2014, was published in the NCCN guidelines; however, as with the ASCO guideline, ovarian tissue cryopreservation was considered experimental and under clinical trial [28]. On the other hand, in 2014, the American Society for Reproductive Medicine (ASRM) committee announced the following opinions with regard to ovarian tissue cryopreservation: (1) Ovarian tissue cryopreservation and transplantation are experimental; (2) Ovarian tissue cryopreservation is an option for patients who require immediate gonadotoxic treatment and may be used for prepubescent girls only; (3) Ovarian tissue cryopreservation should not be provided for patients with benign tumors or in a situation where the patient desires a late pregnancy; (4) Ovarian tissue may be transplanted into a pelvic (orthotopic) or extrapelvic (heterotopic) site; (5) Ovarian tissue in humans has been cryopreserved as cortical biopsies or stripes or as whole ovaries. Human ovarian tissue is preserved as a biopsy of the ovarian cortical tissue, or unilateral ovarian cortex, or bilateral whole ovaries; (6) Ovarian tissue may be transplanted into a pelvic (orthotopic) or extrapelvic (heterotopic) site. Ovarian tissue may be transplanted orthotopically or heterotopically; (7) Pregnancies and live births have been achieved only with orthotopic transplantation of cortical stripes; however, date are confounded by the fact that the pregnancy could have resulted from ovulation from a native ovary; (8) No pregnancies have been reported to date either from thawed ovarian tissue transplanted ovarian tissue transplanted into a heterotopic site or as a result of thawed whole ovary transplantation. In heterotopic transplantation and whole ovary transplantation, there have been no pregnancies reported; (9) Ovarian tissue transplantation carries a potential risk of reintroducing malignancy." [2].

5.3 Ovarian Cortical Tissue Vitrification

As a method of preserving fertility of young women, with fertilized eggs (embryo, blastcyst) or oocytes, it has been said that vitrification, rather than slow freezing, has become common practice for preservation. However, with regard to the preservation methods for ovarian tissue, slow freezing is the standard method. Few facilities perform vitrification as the main preserving method in ovarian tissue freezing, which has been studied since around 2005. Yeoman et al. [29] reported the survival rate of follicles in the ovaries with slow freezing and vitrification in monkey ovaries. According to their report, there was no difference in survival rate of follicles between the slow freezing method and vitrification, and they claimed that in the future, vitrification may be an option of preserving fertility [29]. On the other hand, Gandolfi et al. [30] reported that the best animal model to examine vitrification of ovaries was that of the cow [30]. Furthermore, Ting et al. [31] reported that on comparing vitrification in ovarian tissue freezing with a control group (non-freezing group), no major abnormalities were seen in tissue images on electron microscopy and staining [31]. Keros et al. [32] conducted a comparison of freezing solution concentrations in slow freezing and vitrification using human ovaries. Two freezing solutions were used, i.e., the one for slow freezing principally comprising Pr-OH (Propanediol) and EG (ethylene glycol), and another comprising DMSO (dimethyl sulphoxide), PrOH, and EG. They prepared concentrated preparations of these freezing solutions (twofold concentration, 0.75 M and 1.5 M) and conducted histological evaluation of ovarian tissues that underwent freezing/thawing in these solutions and 24-h culturing. As a result, although no remarkable difference was found in the follicles at the two different concentrations, the stroma in the vitrification method showed better electron microscopy findings [32]. Sheikhi et al. [33] cryopreserved ovarian tissue by vitrification using cryo tubes and human ovaries, and examined the usefulness of a closed ovarian tissue freezing device. With regard to the freezing solution, the solutions reported by Keros et al. namely

PrOH, EG, and DMSO were prepared. Concentrations tested were 2.5 %, 5 %, and 10 %, and 10 % polyvinylpyrrolidon (PVP) was added to the 10 % solution with incubation time set to 5 min, 10 min, and 10 min, respectively, according to the solution concentration gradient. As a result, there was no remarkable change for any solution, and the results were the same as those of the control group [33]. Amorim et al. [34] reported a review of slow freezing and vitrification, in which, based on reports to date by various researchers, the difficulties in comparing slow freezing and vitrification methods have been pointed out (Table 5.1). To be more specific, due to the difference in ovarian morphology, inter-species comparisons are not feasible, and comparative examinations cannot be achieved for differences in multiple factors, such as the constitution of cryopreservation solutions, tissue

Table 5.1 The evaluation of ovarian tissue between slow freezing and vitrification

Measurement	Vitrification is better	No differences	Slowfreezing is better
Histologic evaluation	Wang 2008	Klocke 2015 Herraiz 2014	Gandolfi 2006
		Amorim 2012 Xiao 2010	
		Isachenko 2009 Keros 2009	
		Rahimi 2009	
Follicle population	Herraiz 2014	Klocke 2015	
	Primordial : Amorim 2012	Isachenko 2009	
	Wang 2008	Huang 2008	
Cell death	Amorim 2012	Herraiz 2014	
		Rahini 2004	
		Rahimi 2004	
TUNEL, DAPI		Xiao 2010	
		Huang 2008	
		Li 2007	
Apopoptosis			Rahimi 2009
Cell proliferation and vascularization/proliferation for follicles		Herraiz 2014	
		Amorim 2012	
Fibrosis	Xiao 2010	Herraiz 2014	
	Keros 2009	Amorim 2012	
	Wang 2008	Li 2007	
Tissu viability	Herraiz 2014		Isachenko 2009
GAPDH (PCR)	Xiao 2010		
LDH			
Hormone assay		Klocke 2015 Isachenko 2009	
		Huang 2008	
		Li 2007	

The modified table, from Amorim [34] Vitrification as an alternative

immersion time, the device at the time of cryopreservation, the solution used to thaw the frozen tissue, subsequent time for the tissue cultures, and tissue evaluation methods. There are fewer reports of ovarian tissue cryopreserved using the vitrification method than there are using the slow freezing method, and thus, the evaluation of vitrification is still thought to be inadequate. Finally, it has been noted that the safety and effectiveness according to the use of highly concentrated cryoprotective agent should be examined further [34]. On the other hand, we started to develop a new ovarian tissue vitrification method in 2006 using the ovarian tissue of the cynomolgus monkey, the results of which have been previously reported [35, 36, 38]. We will do an additional explanation for that. We removed the bilateral ovaries of seven healthy parous cynomolgus monkeys (85–137 months old), and the ovarian cortex was frozen after removing the medulla. VSED solution (H199 supplemented with 20 % SSS、3.22 mol/l EG、2.56 mol/l DMSO、0.5 mol/l sucrose) [37] reported by Ishimori et al. [37] was one solution, the other was VSEGP solution (H199 supplemented with 20 % SSS, 5.64 mol/l EG、5 % PVP and 0.5 mol sucrose) [30], and the two were compared. Eventually, VSDGP was used by histological and electron microscope tests [35]. Thereafter, under these conditions, further studies proceeded, and the restoration of the menstrual cycle was confirmed in the transplanted ovaries in the omentum, iliac fossa, and uterine serosa. In the end, viable embryos were successfully obtained three times from two individuals [38]. Thereafter, we started to apply this technique in patients with medical conditions requiring cryopreservation [40, 41]. At present (June 2016), we have cryopreserved ova in 229 cases including POI and cancer patients with this technique since January 2010 (breast cancer, 55 cases; systemic lupus erythematosus (SLE), 4 cases; myelodysplastic syndrome (MDS), 3 cases; cervical cancer (SCC), 2 cases; Ewing sarcoma, 1 case; rectal cancer, 1 case; malignant lymphoma, 1 case; CTLA gene abnomality, 1 case; premature ovarian failure (POI), 161 cases and achieved 2 live births, (both of which were POI patients) [39, 40] and one miscarriage. In most patients, the menstrual cycle was confirmed following transplantation. Presently, the device we use is the open device (Ova cryo Kit Type M ®)). No particular problems have occurred with cryopreservation.

5.4 Whole Ovarian Tissue Vitrification

Revel et al. have studied ovarian tissue vitrification using the whole ovarian tissue of large animals (sheep) in 2004 [42]. Courbiere et al. attempted vitrification of the whole ovarian tissue of sheep in 2005 and reported no abnormalities in histological findings in the vitrification of follicles [43]; however, as a result of subsequent close examination, they reported in 2006 that ovarian tissue freezing by vitrification of the whole ovarian tissue was extremely difficult [44]. The underlying reason is that the location of occurrence of ice formation in the ovary is unknown, and the tissue is affected differently once it has been thawed depending on where ice has formed. When whole ovaries are intended to be transplanted, blood vessels need be retained during freezing and thawing for implantation by vascular anastomosis. However, frozen blood vessels are highly likely to degenerate, leading to major changes in the ovarian tissue following transplantation. On the other hand, if the presence of blood vessels facilitates re-establishment of blood flow and thereby improves the survival rate of thawed ovarian transplant, ovarian functions can be expected to be better maintained through transplantation. In 2009 Courbiere et al. achieved successful offspring birth through the whole ovarian tissue vitrification in sheep; however, they described that there were only few viable follicles remaining in the ovaries, and therefore, further improvements in the process would be necessary [45].

5.5 Clinical Application of Ovarian Cortical Tissue Vitrification

To date, not many reports have described the actual clinical application of ovarian cortical tissue vitrification. Silber et al. froze ovaries using the slow freezing and vitrification methods and reported no problem in hormone balance following thawing and transplantation. Similarly, on performing ovarian tissue freezing by vitrification there was no problem in ischemic interval due to transplantation of freeze-thawed ovaries [46]. Thereafter, in 2013 Kikuchi et al. clinically applied ovarian cortical tissue vitrification and successfully harvested oocytes [47]. They reported that ovarian cortical tissue vitrification to be safe in humans [48]. As mentioned above, we completed pre-clinical tests using cynomolgus monkey and started to clinically apply ovarian tissue vitrification method, a novel ovarian tissue freezing method that we had been developing since January 2010, with the implementation of which, we have successfully achieved live births [40, 41].

5.6 Our Target of Ovarian Cortex Vitrification in St. Marianna University

The ovarian tissue freezing protocols of our hospital, when ovarian tissue vitrification is determined, hospitalization period is in total of 3 days (1 day prior to and 2 days after surgery). In the actual case, the following points are necessary for confirmation when moving into the hospital 1 day prior to the surgery date: menstruation cycle, number of antral follicles inside the ovary, hormone value (FSH, LH, E2, P4, AMH etc.). Then after re-confirming with eyes in SILS (single incision laparoscopic surgery) we operate with the one-side of ovarian excision by bipolar and retrieve the ovary.

5.7 Protocol of Ovarian Tissue Vitrifycation (Figs. 5.1, 5.2, 5.3, 5.4, 5.5, 5.6, and 5.7)

Required Materials
Some dishes
Tweezers
Scissors
Surgical knife
Syringe+Needle
Sterilized gauge
Ova Cryo device Type M and Ova Cryo Kit Type M

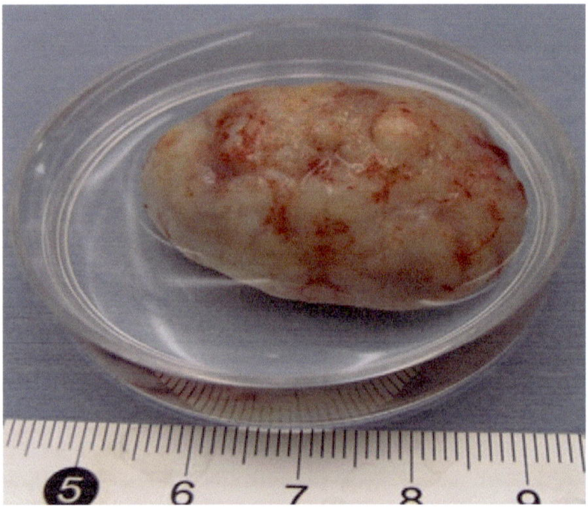

Fig. 5.1 Resection of the ovary

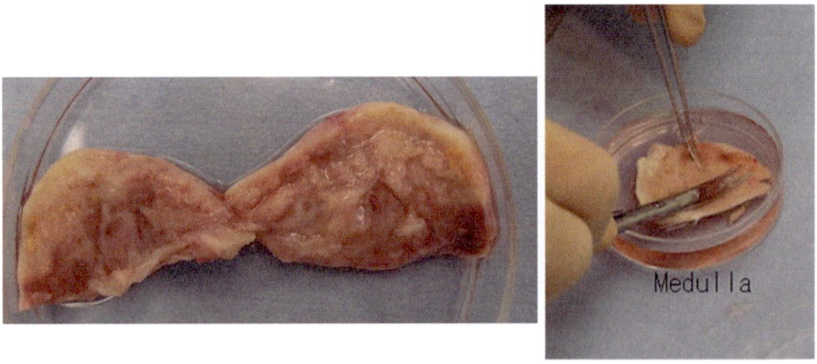

Fig. 5.2 Separation of the medulla

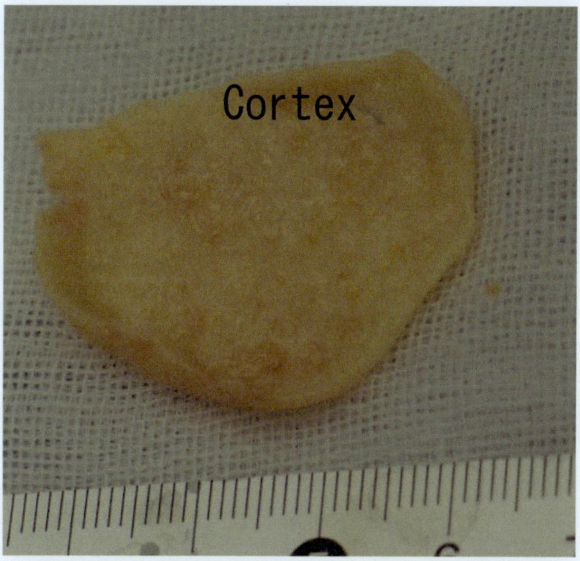

Fig. 5.3 The sheet of cortex

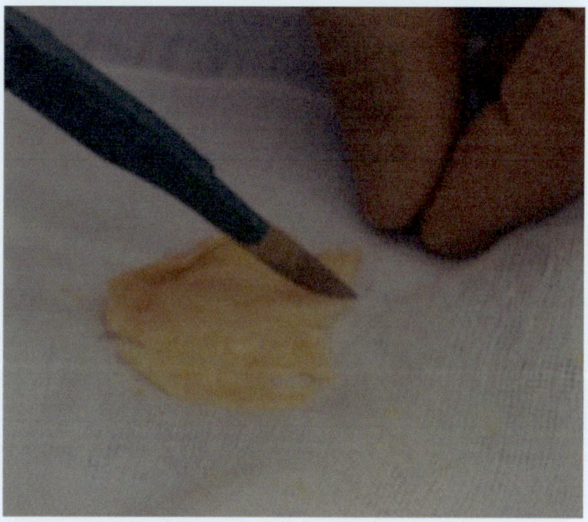

Fig. 5.4 Dicing up the ovarian cortex

1. Wash it with saline to remove blood on the 37 °C warm plate after laparoscopic surgery.
2. Puncture the follicles with a needle and absorb them and collect oocytes.
   After confirming the oocytes, perform IVF.
3. Open the ovary up on the 37°C warm plate.
4. Separate the extra medulla. Only the cortex is left.
5. On a glass laboratory dish, cut the cortex into small pieces (10 × 10 × 1 mm)

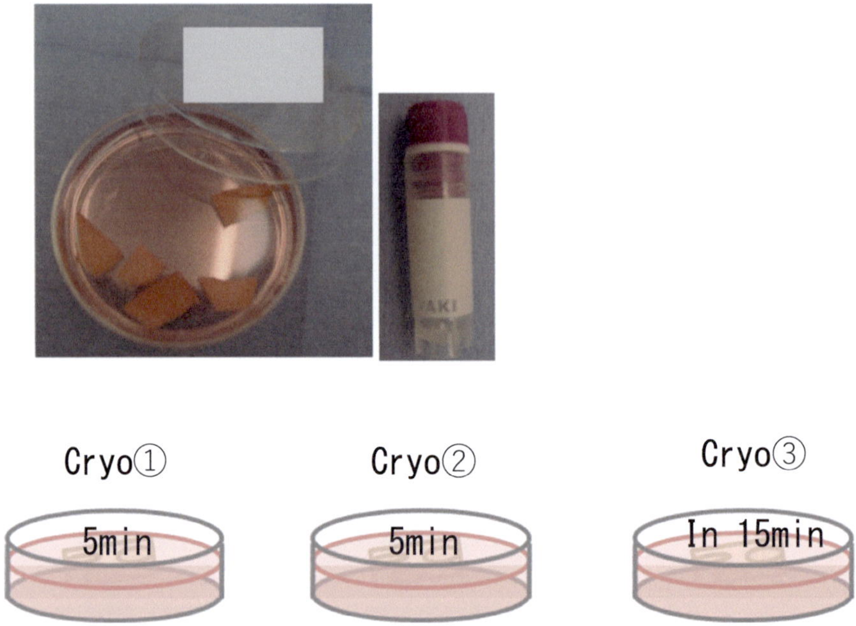

Fig. 5.5 Equilibration of ovarian tissues

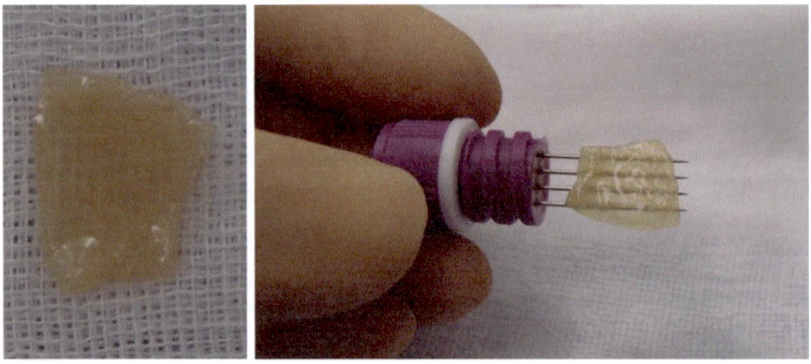

Fig. 5.6 Putting on the tissue

6. Ovarian pieces were equilibrated with three increasing concentrations of cryoprotectants under room temperature such as around 26 °C. Prepare the Type M device and the liquid nitrogen in the meantime.
7. The ovary becomes semitransparent when a freeze reagent is substituted.

   Place the ovarian tissue on the gauze once to remove extra fluid. Mount individual ovarian tissue on the device to allow maximization of its surface area and immerse it in liquid N2 immediately.
8. Cast the device in liquid nitrogen with tweezers so that the device does not detach within the liquid nitrogen.

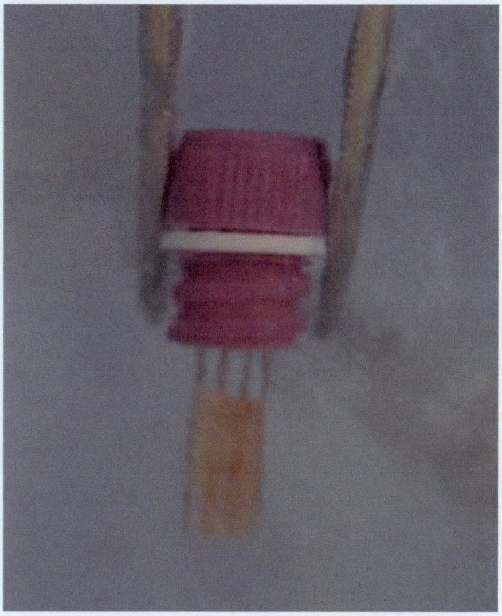

Fig. 5.7 Immersing into liquid nitrogen

5.8 Protocol of Thawing Ovarian Tissue After Vitrifycation (Figs. 5.8, 5.9, 5.10, and 5.11)

Required Materials
Water bath
4.5 oz specimen container
Some dishes
Tweezers
Ova Thawing Kit Type M
10 %SSS+M-HTF 50 ml.

1. Remove the cover of the device in liquid nitrogen and warm a water bath to 37 °C
   And immerse Type M in the thawing liquid quickly in the water bath.
2. Let the ovarian tissue immerse in the fusion liquid for 1 min under 37 °C.
   And shake the type M device lightly so that the ovarian tissue detaches and enters the thawing liquid.
3. One minute later, move the tissue quickly from cup ① to dish ② under 37 °C.
   This works just like the sequential thawing of the embryo.
4. Leave the ovarian tissue in the M-HTF medium prewarmed to 37 °C for 5 min.

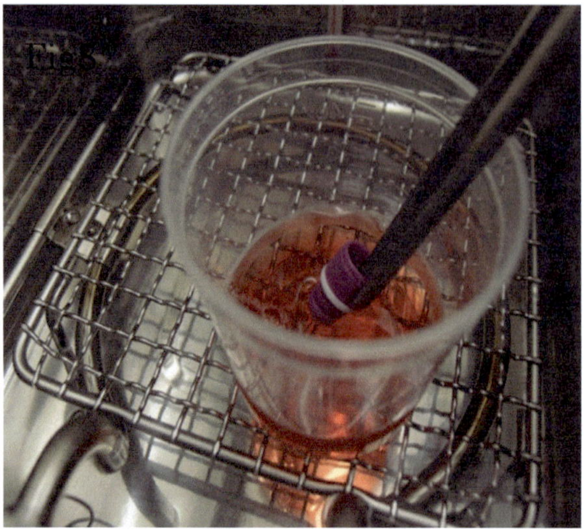

Fig. 5.8 Immersing into thawing medium

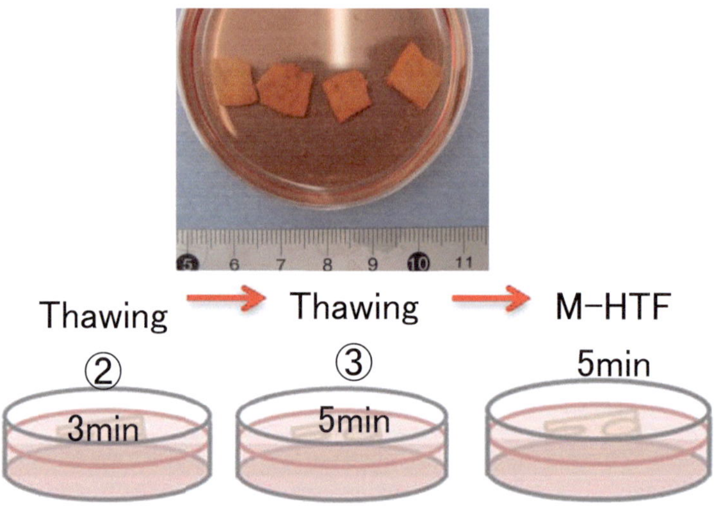

Fig. 5.9 Dilution of cryoprotectant from the tissue

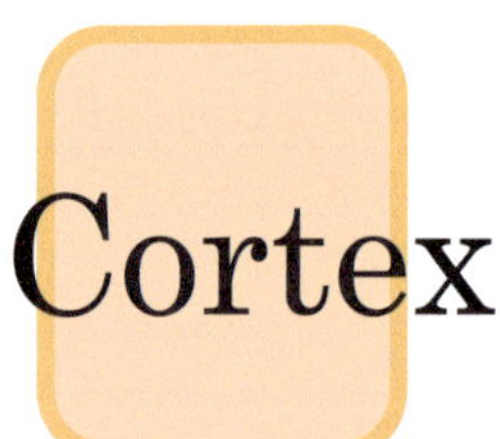

Fig. 5.10 The cortex sheet of ovarian tissue

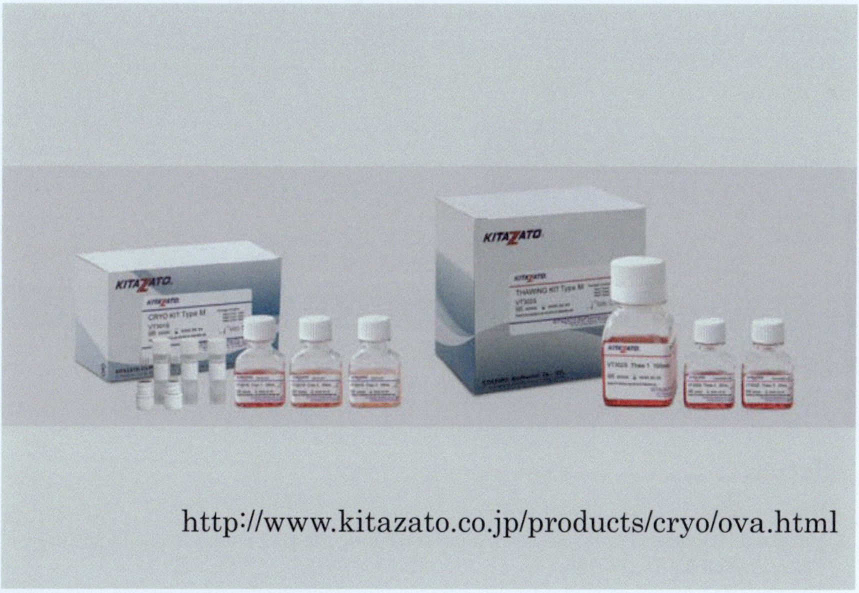

Fig. 5.11 Vitrification device and solutions

5.9 Future Perspective

Bielanski [49] reported that, given the risk of infection in liquid nitrogen, animal tissue that is intended to be preserved for longer durations, including human embryos and tissue, should not be preserved directly in liquid nitrogen. Additionally, to avoid cross-contamination, a seal was required to prevent the tissue from contacting liquid nitrogen directly (depending on the conditions, a double seal was recommended) [49]. While a closed device already exists for human ova and embryos, there are almost no reports of even open devices for human ovarian tissue freezing or of closed devices as a manufactured product. Therefore, we have started to develop a closed device for ovarian tissue freezing. Taking heat conduction efficiency of the device into consideration [39], we measured the condactance of four fine needles (Cryo Support) Hashimoto [35], a copper sheet, and a carbon graphite sheet. We found the carbon graphite sheet to be ideal for making a device with highest heat conduction efficiency (Fig. 5.12: Photographs of carbon graphite sheet device) [39]. However, although carbon graphite sheet has good heat conduction efficiency, from the perspective of its clinical application, hopes have been abandoned for its utilization. A closed ovarian tissue device with materials that satisfy medical standards is under development, and presently, its pre-clinical studies are underway.

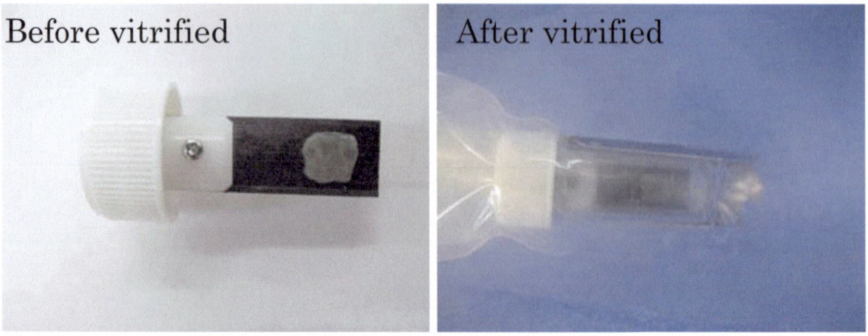

Fig. 5.12 The device of Carbon graphite

References

1. Hoagland H, Pincus G (1942) Revival of mammalian sperm after immersion in liquid nitrogen. J Gen Physiol 25(3):337–344
2. The Practice Committee of the American Society for Reproductive Medicine (2014) Ovarian tissue cryopreservation: a committee opinion. Fertil Steril 101(5):1237–1243
3. Cakmak H, Audra Katz RN, Cedars MI, Rosen MP (2013) Effective method for emergency fertility preservation: random-start controlled ovarian stimulation. Fertil Steril 100 (6):1673–1680
4. Oktay K, Nugent D, Newton H, Salha O, Chatterigee P, Gosden RG (1997) Isolation and characterizeation of primordiall follicles from fresh and cryopreserved human ovarian tissue. Fertil Steril 3:481–486
5. Oktay K, Newton H, Aubanrd Y, Salha O, Gosden RG (1998) Cryopreservation of immature human oocytes and ovarian tissue: an emerging technology? Fertil Steril 59(1):1–7
6. Newthon H, Aubard Y, Rutherford A, Sharma V, Gosden R (1996) Low temperature storage and grafting of human ovarian tissue. Hum Reprod 11(7):1487–1491
7. Hovatta O, Silye R, Krausz T, Abir R, Margara R, Trew G, Lass A, Winston RM (1996) Cryopreservation of human ovarian tissue using dimethylsulphoxide and propanediol-sucrose as cryoprotectants. Hum Reprod 11(6):1268–1272
8. Donnez J, Bassil S (1998) Indications of cryopreservation of ovarian tissue. Hum Reprod Update 4(3):248–259
9. Meirow D, Ben Yehuda D, Prus D, Poliack A, Schenker JG, Rachmilewiz EA, Lewin A (1998) Ovarian tissue banking in patients with Hodgkin's disease: is it safe? Fertil Steril 69 (6):996–998
10. Oktay K, Buyuk E, Veeck L, Zaninovic N, Xu K, Takeuchi T, Opsahl M, Rosenwaks Z (2004) Embryo development after heterotopic transplantation of cryopreserved ovarian tissue. Lancet 363:837–840
11. Donnez J, Dolmans MM, Demylle D, Jadoul P, Pirard C, Squifflet J, Martinez-Madrid B, Van Langendonckt A (2004) Livebirth after orthotopic transplantation of cryopreserved ovarian tissue. Lancet 364:1405–1410
12. Callejo J, Salvador C, Miralles A et al (2001) Long-term ovarian function evaluation after autografting by implantation with fresh and frozen–thawed human ovarian tissue. J Clin Endocrinol Metab 8:4489–4494
13. Fabbri R (2006) Cryopreservation of human oocytes and ovarian tissue. Cell Tissue Bank 7:113–122

14. Gook DA, McCully BA, Edgar DH, McBain JC (2001) Development of antral follicles in human cryopreserved ovarian tissue following xenografting. Hum Reprod 16:417–422
15. Gook DA, Edgar DH, Borg J et al (2003) Oocyte maturation, follicle rupture and luteinization in human cryopreserved ovar- ian tissue following xenografting. Hum Reprod 18:1772–1781
16. Gook DA, Edgar DH, Borg J et al (2005) Diagnostic assess- ment of the developmental potential of human cryopreserved ovarian tissue from multiple patients using xenografting. Hum Reprod 26:72–78
17. Kim SS, Hwang IT, Lee HC, Kim DH (2003) Ovarian function after autotransplantation of frozen thawed human ovarian tissue: an experience of human ovarian grafting into two eterotopic sites. Fertil Steril 80:94–95
18. Kim SS, Hwang IT, Lee HC (2004) Heterotopic autotrans- plantation of cryobanked human ovarian tissue as a strategy to restore ovarian function. Fertil Steril 82:930–932
19. Kim SS, Lee WS, Chung MK et al (2009) Long-term ovarian function and fertility after heterotopic autotransplantation of cryobanked human ovarian tissue: 8-year experience in cancer patients. Fertil Steril 91:2349–2354
20. Meirow D, Levron J, Eldar-Geva T et al (2005) Pregnancy after transplantation of cryopreserved ovarian tissue in a patient with ovarian failure after chemotherapy. N Engl J Med 353:318–321
21. Meirow D, Levron J, Eldar-Geva T et al (2007) Monitoring the ovaries after autotransplantation of cryopreserved ovarian tissue: endocrine studies, in vitro fertilization cycles, and live birth. Fertil Steril 87:418.e7–418.e15
22. Von Wolff M, Donnez J, Hovatta O et al (2009) Cryopreserva- tion and autotransplantation of human ovarian tissue prior to cytotoxic therapy – a technique in its infancy but already successful in fertility preservation. Eur J Cancer 45:1547–1553
23. Stoop D, Cobo A, Silber S (2014) Fertility preservation for age-related fertileity decline. Lancet 384:1311–1319
24. Donnez J, Dolmans MM, Pellicer A, Diaz-Garcia C, Ernst E, Macklon KT, Andersen CY (2015) Fertility preservation for age-related fertility decline. Lancet 385:506–507
25. von Wolff M, Montag M, Dittrich R, Denshlag D, Nawroth F, Lawrenz B (2011) Fertility preservation in women-a practiceal guide to preservation techniques and therapeutic strategyes in breast cancer, Hodgkin's lymphoma and borderline ovaryian tumors by the fertility preservation network FertiPROTEKT. Arch Gynecol Obstet 284:427–435
26. ISFP Practiee Committee, Kim SS, Donnez J, Barri P, Pellicer A, Pasquale P, Rosenwaks Z, Nagy P, Falcone T, Andersen C, Hovatta O, Wallace H, Meirow D, Gook D, Kim SH, Tzeng C-R, Suzuki S, Ishizuka B, Dolmans M-M (2012) Recommendations for fertileity preservation in patients with lymphoma, leukemia, and breast cancer. J Assist Reprod Genet 29:465–468
27. Loren AW, Mangu PB, Beck LN, Brennan L, Magdalinski AJ, Partridge AH, Quinn G, Wallace WH, Oktay K (2013) Fertility preservation for patients with cancer: American Society of Clinical Oncology Clinical Practice Guideline Update. J Clin Oncol 311(19):2500–2511
28. Featured Update to the NCCN Guidelines (2014) Adolescent and Young Adult Oncology, Ver 2.2014. J Natl Compr Cancer Netw. 12(1):21–32
29. Yeoman RR, Wolf DP, Lee DM (2005) Coculture of monkey ovarian tissue increases survival after vitrification and slow-rate freezing. Fertil Steril 83:1248–1254
30. Gandolfi F, Paffoni A, Papasso Brambilla E, Bonetti S, Brevini TAL, Pharm D, Ragni G (2006) Efficiency of equilibrium cooling and vitrification procedures for the cryopreservation of ovarian tissue: comparative analysis between human and animal models. Fertil Steril 85 (1):1150–1156
31. Ting AY, Yeoman RR, Lawson S, Zelinski MB (2011) In vitro development of secondary follicles from cryopreserved rhesus macaque ovarian tissue after slow-rate-freeze or vitrification. Hum Reprod 26(9):2461–2472
32. Keros V, Xella S, Hultenby K, Pettersson K, Sheikhi M, Volpe A, Hreinsson J, Hovatta O (2009) Vitrification versus controlled-rate freezing in cryopreserveation of human ovarian tissue. Hum Reprod 24(7):1670–1683

33. Sheikhi M, Hultendby K, Niklasson B, Lundqvist M, Hobatta O (2011) Clinical grade vitrification: an ultrastructural analysis of follicles and stroma in vitrified tissue. Hum Reprod 26(3):594–603
34. Amorim CA, Curaba M, Van Langendonckt A, Dolmans M-M, Donnez J (2011) Vitrification as analternative means of cryopreserveing ovarian tissue. Repro Biomed On 23:160–186
35. Hashimoto S, Suzuki N, Yamanaka M, Hosoi Y, Ishizuka B, Morimoto Y (2010) Effects of vitrification solutions and equilibrateon times on the morphology of cynomolgus ovaryan tissue. Repro Bio Online 21:501–509
36. Igarashi S, Suzuki N, Hashimoto S, Takae S, Takenoshita M, Hosoi Y, Morimoto Y, Ishizuka B (2010) Heterotopic autotransplantation of ovarian cortex in cynomolgus monkeys. Hum Cell 23(1):26–34
37. Ishimori H, Takahashi Y, Kanagawa H (1992) Factors affecting survival of mouse blastocysts vitrified by a mixture of ethylene glycol and dimethyl sulfoxide. Theriogenology 38:1175–1185
38. Suzuki N, Hashimoto S, Igarashi S, Takae S, Yamanaka M, Yamochi T, Takenosita M, Hosoi Y, Morimoto Y, Ishizuka B (2012) Assesment of long-term function of heterotopic transplants of vitrified ovarian tissue in cynomolgus monkeys. Hum Reprod 27(8):2420–2429
39. Hashimoto S, Suzuki N, Amo A, Yamochi T, Hosoi Y, Morimoto Y (2013) Good thermally conducting material supports follicle morphologyes of procine ovaries cryopreserved with ultrarapid vitrifycation. J Reprod Dev 59(5):496–499
40. Kawamura K, Cheng Y, Suzuki N, Deguchi M, Sato Y, Takae S, Ho CH, Kawamura N, Tamura M, Hashimoto S, Sugishita Y, Morimoto Y, Hosoi Y, Yoshioka N, Ishizuka B, Hsueh AJ (2013) Hippo signaling disruption and Akt stimulation of ovarian follicles for infertility treatment. Proc Natl Acad Sci 110(43):17474–17479
41. Suzuki N, Yoshioka N, Takae S, Sugishita Y, Tamura M, Hashimoto S, Morimoto Y, Kawamura K (2015) Successful fertility preservation following ovarian tissue vitrification in patients with primary ovarian insufficiency. Hum Reprod 30:608–615
42. Revel A, Elami A, Bor A, Yavin S, Natan Y, Arav A (2004) Whole sheep ovary cryopreservation and transplantation. Fertil Steril 82:1714–1715
43. Courbiere B, Massardier J, Salle B, Mazoyer C, Guerin JF, Lornage J (2005) Follicular viability and histological assessment after cryopreservation of whole sheep ovaries with vascular pedicle by vitrification. Fertil Steril 84:1065–1071
44. Courbiere B, Odagescu V, Baudot A, Massardier J, Mazoyer C, Salle B, Lornage J (2006) Cryopreservation of the ovary by vitrification as an alternative to slow-cooling protocols. Fertil Steril 86:1243–1251
45. Courbiere B, Caquant L, Mazoyer C, Franck M, Lornage J, Salle B (2009) Difficulties improving ovarian functional recovery by microvascular transplantation and whole ovary vitrification. Fertil Steril 91:2697–2706
46. Silber S, Kagawa N, Kuwayama M, Gosden R (2010) Duration of fertileity after fresh and frozen ovary transplantation. Fertil Steril 94:2191–2196
47. Kikuchi I, Kagawa N, Silber S, Kuwayama M, Takehara Y, Aono F, Kumakiri J, Kato O, Takeda S (2013) Oophorectomy for fertility preservation via reduced-port laparoscopic surgery. Surg Innov 20(3):219–224
48. Kagawa N, Kikuchi I, Kuwayama M (2015) Ovarian tissue vitrification for fertility preservation. Vitrification in Assisted Reproduction-Springer. 43–49
49. Bielanski A (2014) Biosafety embryo and semen cryopreservation, storage, management and transport. Adv Exp Med Biol 753:429–465

Chapter 6
Ovarian Tissue Freezing and Transplantation: Current Status

Jacques Donnez and Marie-Madeleine Dolmans

Abstract Purpose of Review To carefully evaluate a number of critical points related to ovarian tissue freezing and present factual data in terms of live birth rates and risks.

Recent Findings Reimplantation of frozen-thawed ovarian tissue remains an experimental procedure according to the ASRM, despite more than 40 live births reported in the literature.

Summary This manuscript emphasizes the crucial importance of not only pre serving fertility in young women, but also clearly explaining to patients the different available options and their respective success rates.

Some previously published reviews have reported inaccurate reimplantation success rates. In this review, we report the true picture, with a live birth rate of 25 %.

Ovarian tissue freezing may be combined with pickup of immature oocytes (at the time of ovarian biopsy and tissue removal) or mature oocytes (if chemotherapy can be delayed).

Keywords Ovary • Ovarian tissue cryopreservation • Freezing • Reimplantation

6.1 Introduction

Thanks to advances in cancer therapy over the past two decades, overall rates of death attributable to cancer in women have fallen by >1.6 % per year during the last 5 years [1, 2]. Unfortunately, treatments such as chemotherapy, radiotherapy, and/or surgery can induce premature ovarian failure (POF) in some circumstances [2, 3]. Indeed, the ovaries are very sensitive to cytotoxic drugs, especially alkylating

J. Donnez (✉)
Infertility Research Unit, Société de Recherche pour l'Infertilité (SRI), Av. Grandchamp, 143, 1150 Brussels, Belgium
e-mail: jacques.donnez@gmail.com

M.-M. Dolmans
Gynecology Research Unit, Institut de Recherche Expérimentale et Clinique, Université Catholique de Louvain, Brussels, Belgium

N. Suzuki, J. Donnez (eds.), *Gonadal Tissue Cryopreservation in Fertility Preservation*, DOI 10.1007/978-4-431-55963-4_6

agents and pelvic radiation (exposure to 5–10 Gy) [4], which are likely to cause gonadal dysfunction [5–13]. Cyclophosphamide is the alkylating agent that causes most damage to oocytes and granulosa cells in a dose-dependent manner [5–9].

Giving a patient an accurate assessment of the risk to fertility is very difficult, as how a disease will develop cannot be predicted [10]. Hence, evaluating the likelihood of POF after chemo- or radiotherapy in young cancer patients is often extremely problematic [10, 11].

Benign systemic diseases such as autoimmune and hematological conditions sometimes also require chemo- or radiotherapy, associated with bone marrow transplantation [9, 10]. This treatment combination puts patients at the greatest risk of POF, estimated to be 92–100 % [3, 12], which is mostly related to the use of total body irradiation prior to transplantation and increased age at the time of treatment.

In addition, women are increasingly postponing childbearing to later in life for social or financial reasons, and the incidence of most cancers rises with age [2, 3, 13, 14].

This chapter evaluates the current status of ovarian tissue freezing for fertility preservation purposes.

6.2 Different Options for Fertility Preservation (Fig. 6.1)

Women with cancer have several options to preserve their fertility and enable them to conceive when they have recovered: ovarian transposition, embryo cryopreservation, immature or mature oocyte cryopreservation, and ovarian tissue cryopreservation [13–15]. Currently, embryo and mature oocyte cryopreservation following in vitro fertilization (IVF) are the only methods endorsed by the American Society for Reproductive Medicine (ASRM).

6.3 Ovarian Tissue Cryopreservation

Cryopreservation of ovarian tissue is the only fertility preservation option available to prepubertal girls and women who cannot delay the start of chemotherapy and a specific issue in children. A number of investigators have addressed the question of ovarian tissue freezing during childhood and adolescence, but only a few series have been documented [2, 3, 14]. As recently reviewed [33], research into personalizing the approach to care is critical if we are to meet the needs of this patient population.

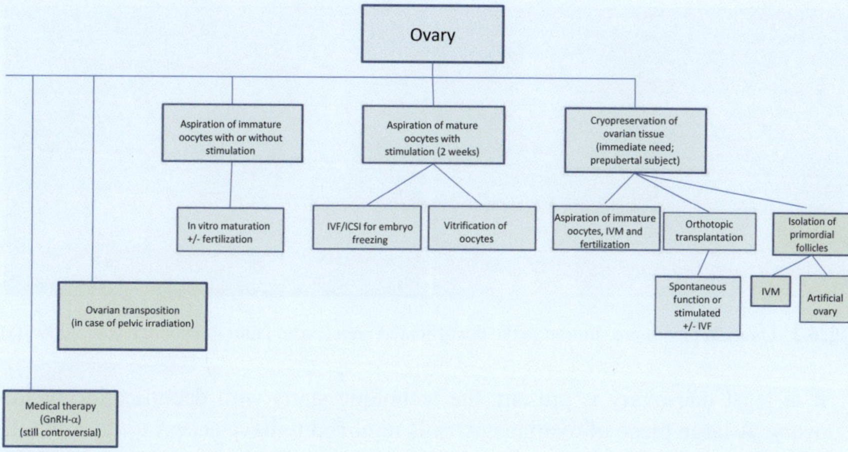

Fig. 6.1 Fertility preservation methods in women at risk of POF. Depending on patient age and possible delay before starting chemotherapy, options include medical therapy to protect the ovaries from chemotherapy (still controversial), ovarian transposition before pelvic radiotherapy, immature oocyte retrieval followed by IVM, mature oocyte retrieval followed by fertilization and embryo freezing or oocyte vitrification, or ovarian tissue cryopreservation. At the time of ovarian tissue cryopreservation, immature oocytes can also be retrieved. After thawing of ovarian tissue, orthotopic transplantation is currently the goal in clinical practice. Indeed, isolation of primordial follicles is still at the research stage. *Abbreviations*: *ICSI* intracytoplasmic sperm injection, *IVF* in vitro fertilization (From Nat. Rev End., 2013 [2])

6.3.1 How Much Ovarian Cortex Should Be Harvested for Cryopreservation?

This decision is influenced mainly by the estimated risk of POF relative to the planned treatment and existing ovarian volume. Oophorectomy should be performed in patients undergoing pelvic irradiation or total body irradiation and in those receiving high doses of alkylating agents. This procedure should also be performed in very young girls (namely prepubertal girls) because of the small size of their ovaries. Otherwise, in adults, four to five ovarian cortical biopsy samples of ~1 cm in length, 4–5 mm in width, and 1.0–1.5 mm in depth are taken in most departments around the world [2, 3], although left oophorectomy is carried out almost systematically in some countries [16].

6.3.2 Techniques of Orthotopic Autotransplantation

Two techniques may be used depending on the presence or not of at least one remaining ovary:

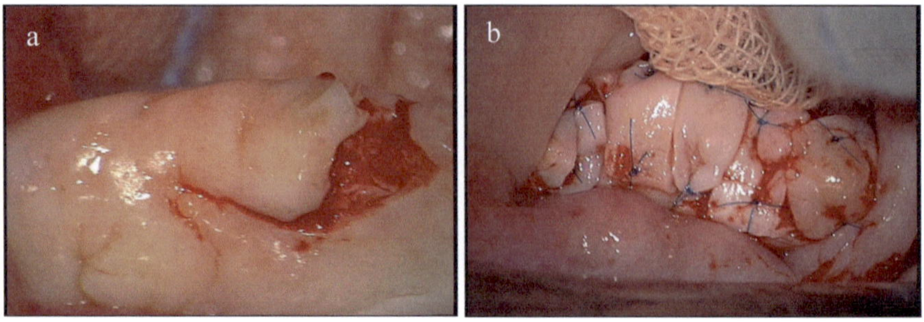

Fig. 6.2 Ovarian pieces are sutured to the decorticated area (From Hum Reprod Update, 2006 [1])

1. If at least one ovary is present, the technique starts with decortication of the ovary. A large piece of ovarian cortex is removed to have access to the medulla (Fig. 6.2) and its vascular network. According to microsurgical techniques, ovarian cortical pieces are then fixed with the use of 7-0 or 8-0 propylene stitches [1, 3, 4], or simply placed on the medulla and fixed with Interceed or fibrin glue. In the series published by Andersen's group [16], ovarian tissue is deposited on the medulla after making an incision in the cortex; the tissue is thus placed in a subcortical area.
2. If both ovaries are absent, a peritoneal window may be created in two steps, as in the case published in 2004 [17], to induce angiogenesis before the grafting procedure, or in one step, as recently described [31]. The incision for this peritoneal window is made on the anterior leaf of the broad ligament in an area where a vascular network is visible (retroperitoneal vessels, Fig. 6.3). The fragments are placed in the window and subsequently covered with Interceed, the edges of which are fixed with fibrin glue. The peritoneal window method may also be applied if a nonfunctional ovary is still in place.

6.3.3 Restoration of Ovarian Activity

In a series of 60 cases of frozen-thawed ovarian tissue reimplantation, restoration of ovarian activity was observed in all cases but three, where no follicles were present in the reimplanted tissue, highlighting the importance of evaluating follicular density before making the decision to reimplant [14]. In this series (including Danish, Spanish and Belgian teams), the peritoneal window created close to the ovarian hilus and the ovarian medulla both proved to be equally efficient sites, at least for restoration of ovarian activity (as evidenced by follicular development and circulating steroid levels). Large strips (8–10 × 5 mm) and small cubes (2 mm^3) of tissue were also both shown to effectively restore ovarian endocrine function.

In all instances, it took 3.5–6.5 months after reimplantation before an increase in estradiol (E2) and a decrease in follicle-stimulating hormone (FSH) were detected (mean 4.5 months). The time interval between implantation of cortical tissue and

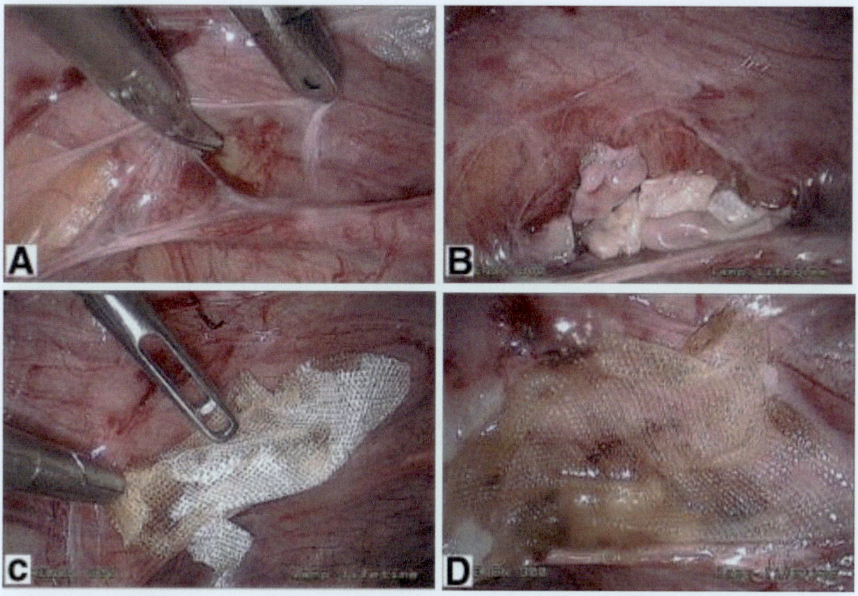

Fig. 6.3 Surgical procedure. **a** Creation of the peritoneal window in the anterior leaf of the broad ligament. **b** Cryopreserved-thawed ovarian fragments are placed in the peritoneal window. **c**, **d** The pieces of ovarian cortex are then covered with Interceed (From Fertil. Steril. 2012 [17])

the first E2 peak is consistent with data obtained from sheep and humans, although some variation may be observed [28] and explained by a difference in follicular reserve at the time of cryopreservation (Fig. 6.3).

In our opinion, the pelvic cavity (orthotopic site) provides the optimal environment for follicular development compared with heterotopic sites, as temperature, pressure, paracrine factors, and blood supply are similar to those observed in a physiological situation. Even if transplanting ovarian tissue to heterotopic sites has some advantages [18, 19], only one pregnancy has been reported following this procedure [20], making this approach somewhat questionable [14].

6.4 Restoration of Ovarian Activity and Live Birth Rate

The number of women undergoing reimplantations worldwide (the denominator) is not known. In 2013, results from three centers (in Denmark, Spain and Belgium) were collected to evaluate a series of 60 cases of orthotopic reimplantation [14]. Restoration of ovarian activity was observed in 93 % of patients and the pregnancy rate was 25 %. An absence of primordial follicles in the reimplanted tissue explains the lack of postgrafting ovarian activity in the remaining 7 % [1]. The mean duration of ovarian function after transplantation is normally ~4–5 years [2, 3].

6.4.1 The True Picture

In the light of growing interest in fertility preservation, we feel it is time to carefully evaluate all currently available options to preserve fertility in female cancer patients and women at risk of POF. It is also necessary to amend some misleading information that appeared in a very recent paper [21], in which data presented in the tables were confused and inaccurate, as numbers of reported cases and pregnancies did not correspond to those published in the literature. Moreover, the exact number of transplants was unknown, yielding erroneous pregnancy and live birth rates. Many of the cases were simply case reports, making any interpretation unreliable.

Only existing data documented in peer-reviewed journals, an analysis of which was recently published, should be taken into account and reviewed [22]. To date, 60 live births have been reported in peer-reviewed journals (Table 6.1). It is important to stress that only published live births can be included in this analysis. A hypothetical number resulting from phone calls to different centers is in no way representative of the facts.

Table 6.1 Series of 60 live births after transplantation of frozen-thawed ovarian cortex

	Cryopreservation procedure	Number of transplanted women desiring pregnancy	Number of live births (..)=ongoing pregnancies
Donnez, Dolmans et al.	SF	19	8 (+1)
Meirow et al.	SF	NA	6
Demeestere et al.	SF	NA	3
Andersen et al.	SF	25	8
Silber et al.	SF	6	4
Piver et al., Roux et al.	SF	NA	3 (+1)
Pellicer et al.	SF	33	6[a] (+3)
Revel et al.	SF	NA	2
Dittrich et al.	SF	20	6
Revelli et al.	SF	NA	1
Callejo et al.	SF	NA	1
Stern, Gook, Rozen	SF	14	3[a]
Kawamura, Suzuki et al.	VF	NA	2
Burmeister, Kovacs, et al.	SF	2	1
Rodriguez-Wallberg, Hovatta et al.	SF	NA	1
Tanbo et al.	SF	2	2
Agarwal et al.[b]	SF	NA	1
Makolkin et al., Kalugina et al.[b]	SF	NA	2

Adapted from The Lancet [22] and from JARG [26]
SF Slow freezing, *VF* Vitrification
[a]twins
[b]Personal communication

Table 6.2 Results from four centers, allowing evaluation of pregnancy and live birth rates, as the number of transplants is known

Teams	Number of transplanted women	Women who conceived	Women who gave birth	Number of live births	Miscarriages
Donnez, Dolmans team	13	3	3	6[a, b]	
Andersen, Macklon team	25	6	4	6[a, b]	2
Pellicer team	22	4	3	4	1
Dittrich team	20	7	4 (+2[c])	4 (+2[c])	1
	80	20 (25 %)	14	20	

From the Lancet [22]
[a]One woman delivered twice
[b]One woman delivered three times
[c]Two ongoing pregnancies

Since publication of these data in the Lancet, two more papers by Rodriguez-Wallberg et al. and Suzuki et al. [23, 24]. Moreover, the first live birth achieved by the Australian team of Kovacs should be added [25] (Table 1 from Donnez et al. JARG, 2015).

As previously stated, pregnancy and live birth rates cannot be extrapolated from case reports, as the denominator is unknown. To set the record straight, results from four centers (in Denmark, Spain, Belgium and Germany), including two very recent series [26, 27], were combined, totaling 80 cases in all (Table 6.2). These results provide a clear and accurate picture of existing pregnancy and live birth rates.

In this series of 80 cases, the pregnancy rate, expressed as the number of women who conceived, is 25 % (20/80), and the number of women who gave birth is 16. As some women delivered twice or three times after transplantation, the number of live births cannot be used as the numerator. Only the number of women who gave birth can be used as the numerator, while the number of transplanted women is the denominator. In a more recent series (111 cases) the pregnancy rate is 29 % [28].

6.4.2 The Future: Combined Procedure

In the future, cryopreservation of ovarian tissue might be associated with removal of small antral follicles followed by in vitro maturation (IVM). Immature oocytes can also be collected from antral follicles in ovarian tissue at the time of the cryopreservation procedure, matured in vitro and then cryopreserved [29–31]. Indeed, for half of the patients who underwent ovarian tissue cryopreservation, this combined procedure offered an additional chance of becoming pregnant. The first live birth resulting from a cryopreserved embryo obtained from in vitro-matured oocytes collected after oophorectomy was recently reported [30], as was the second clinical pregnancy [31].

On the other hand, as recently published by Dolmans et al., controlled ovarian stimulation for pickup of mature oocytes [32] could be performed immediately after removal of ovarian tissue for freezing, without any adverse effects on the number of oocytes or embryos. Indeed, cryopreservation of the bilateral ovarian cortex followed by IVF treatment is a feasible and safe approach to preserve fertility before oncological treatment. The number of cryopreserved embryos obtained was not statistically different from the control group and not affected by the previous bilateral biopsy carried out for cryopreservation purposes. Moreover, this combined technique does not delay further oncological treatment. It may even be proposed to patients without a male partner in association with oocyte vitrification.

6.5 How to Improve the Results

Dysfunctional folliculogenesis has been described [33] and attributed to (1) asynchrony between granulosa cells and oocyte maturation [34], (2) a reduced ovarian reserve after grafting [2], (3) the delay that occurs before efficient graft revascularization [35], and (4) specific postgrafting activation.

Ischemia is responsible for loss of follicles, as the graft needs 4–5 days to be reoxygenated [35]. Ischemia and oxidative stress may be reduced by using drugs to stimulate revascularization of the graft (such as vascular endothelial growth factor (VEGF) or sphingosine-1-phosphate [S1P]) or some inhibitory hormones (e.g. anti-Müllerian hormone [AMH]) that normally operate in an intact ovary.

Another mechanism by which remaining follicles are overactivated due to the lack of AMH could also be implicated [36, 37]. AMH present in growing follicles after transplantation is able to act as a "brake" on initial follicular activation (occurring immediately after transplantation) [35], thereby protecting the pool of residual primordial follicles.

The concept of the vascular bed is therefore important in this regard. It involves preparing the host vascular bed prior to grafting by addition of encapsulated VEGF [38] or stromal cells enriched in CD34, for example, and represents one principal means of improving graft revascularization [39].

In conclusion, more than 40 live births have so far been reported in peer-reviewed journals. It is time to stop considering this procedure as experimental.

References

1. Donnez J, Martinez-Madrid B, Jadoul P et al (2006) Ovarian tissue cryopreservation and transplantation: a review. Hum Reprod Update 12:519–535
2. Donnez J, Dolmans MM (2013) Fertility preservation in women. Nat Rev Endocrinol 9:735–749
3. Donnez J, Dolmans MM (2014) Transplantation of ovarian tissue. Best Pract Res Clin Obstet Gynaecol 28:1188–1197

4. Wallace WH, Thomson AB, Kelsey TW (2003) The radiosensitivity of the human oocyte. Hum Reprod 18:117–121
5. Wallace WHB, Anderson RA, Irvine DS (2005) Fertility preservation for young patients with cancer: who is at risk and what can be offered? Lancet Oncol 6:209–219
6. Meirow D, Nugent D (2001) The effects of radiotherapy and chemotherapy on female reproduction. Hum Reprod Update 7:535–543
7. Donnez J, Dolmans MM, Demylle D et al (2006) Restoration of ovarian function after orthotopic (intraovarian and periovarian) transplantation of cryopreserved ovarian tissue in a woman treated by bone marrow transplantation for sickle cell anemia: case report. Hum Reprod 21:183–188
8. Wallace WH, Thomson AB, Saran F, Kelsey TW (2005) Predicting age of ovarian failure after radiation to a field that includes the ovaries. Int J Radiat Oncol Biol Phys 62:738–744
9. Jadoul P, Donnez J (2012) How does bone marrow transplantation affect ovarian function and fertility? Curr Opin Obstet Gynecol 24:164–171
10. Jadoul P, Dolmans MM, Donnez J (2010) Fertility preservation in girls during childhood: is it feasible, efficient and safe and to whom should it be proposed? Hum Reprod Update 16:617–630
11. Wallace WH, Smith AG, Kelsey TW et al (2014) Fertility preservation for girls and young women with cancer: population-based validation of criteria for ovarian tissue cryopreservation. Lancet Oncol 15:1129–1136
12. Teinturier C, Hartmann O, Valteau-Couanet D et al (1998) Ovarian function after autologous bone marrow transplantation in childhood: high-dose busulfan is a major cause of ovarian failure. Bone Marrow Transplant 22:989–994
13. Bedoschi G, Oktay K (2013) Current approach to fertility preservation by embryo cryopreservation. Fertil Steril 99:1496–1502
14. Cobo A, Garcia-Velasco JA, Domingo J et al (2013) Is vitrification of oocytes useful for fertility preservation for age-related fertility decline and in cancer patients? Fertil Steril 99:1485–1495
15. Cakmak H, Rosen MP (2013) Ovarian stimulation in cancer patients. Fertil Steril 99:1476–1484
16. Andersen CY, Rosendahl M, Byskov AG et al (2008) Two successful pregnancies following autotransplantation of frozen/thawed ovarian tissue. Hum Reprod 23:2266–2272
17. Donnez J, Jadoul P, Pirard C et al (2012) Live birth after transplantation of frozen-thawed ovarian tissue after bilateral oophorectomy for benign disease. Fertil Steril 98:720–725
18. Oktay K, Economos K, Kan M et al (2001) Endocrine function and oocyte retrieval after autologous transplantation of ovarian cortical strips to the forearm. JAMA 26:1490–1493
19. Kim SS (2012) Assessment of long term endocrine function after transplantation of frozen-thawed human ovarian tissue to the heterotopic site: 10 year longitudinal follow-up study. J Assist Reprod Genet 29:489–493
20. Stern CJ, Gook D, Hale LG et al (2013) First reported clinical pregnancy following heterotopic grafting of cryopreserved ovarian tissue in a woman after a bilateral oophorectomy. Hum Reprod 28:2996–2999
21. Stoop D, Cobo A, Silber S (2014) Fertility preservation for age-related fertility decline. Lancet 384(9950):1311–1319
22. Donnez J, Dolmans MM, Pellicer A et al (2015) Fertility preservation for age-related fertility decline. Lancet Letter to the Editor 385(9967):506–507
23. Rodriguez-Wallberg KA, Karlström PO et al (2015) Full-term newborn after repeated ovarian tissue transplants in a patient treated for Ewing sarcoma by sterilizing pelvic irradiation and chemotherapy. Acta Obstet Gynecol Scand 94(3):324–328
24. Suzuki N, Yoshioka N, Takae S, Sugishita Y, Tamura M, Hashimoto S, Morimoto Y, Kawamura K (2015) Successful fertility preservation following ovarian tissue vitrification in patients with primary ovarian insufficiency. Hum Reprod 30(3):608–615

25. Burmeister L, Kovacs GT, Osianlis T (2013) First Australian pregnancy after ovarian tissue cryopreservation and subsequent autotransplantation. Med J Aust 198(3):158–159
26. Donnez J, Dolmans MM (2015) Ovarian cortex transplantation: 60 reported live births brings the success and worldwide expansion of the technique towards routine clinical practice. J Assist Reprod Genet 32(8):1167–1170
27. Dittrich R, Hackl J, Lotz L et al (2015) Pregnancies and live births after 20 transplantations of cryopreserved ovarian tissue in a single center. Fertil Steril 103(2):462–468. doi:10.1016/j.fertnstert.2014.10.045
28. Donnez J, Dolmans MM, Diaz C, Pellicer A (2015) Ovarian cortex transplantation: time to move on from experimental studies to open clinical application. Fertil Steril 104(5):1097–1098
29. Fasano G, Moffa F, Dechène J et al (2011) Vitrification of in vitro matured oocytes collected from antral follicles at the time of ovarian tissue cryopreservation. Reprod Biol Endocrinol 9:150
30. Prasath EB, Chan ML, Wong WH et al (2014) First pregnancy and live birth resulting from cryopreserved embryos obtained from in vitro matured oocytes after oophorectomy in an ovarian cancer patient. Hum Reprod 29:276–278
31. Segers I, Mateizel I, Guzman L, et al (2015) In vitro maturation of ex vivo harvested oocytes obtained after ovariectomy: a promising additional source of gamete preservation leading to the first clinical pregnancy in UZ Brussel. In: Proceedings of the Congress "Freezing of oocytes, embryos and ovarian tissue: focus on fertility management and fertility preservation. Brussels, 16–17 January 2015. JARG, submitted
32. Dolmans MM, Marotta ML, Pirard C et al (2014) Ovarian tissue cryopreservation followed by controlled ovarian stimulation and pick-up of mature oocytes does not impair the number or quality of retrieved oocytes. J Ovarian Res 7:80
33. Dolmans MM, Donnez J, Camboni A et al (2009) IVF outcome in patients with orthotopically transplanted ovarian tissue. Hum Reprod 24:2778–2787
34. Nottola SA, Camboni A, Van Langendonckt A et al (2008) Cryopreservation and xenotransplantation of human ovarian tissue: an ultrastructural study. Fertil Steril 90:23–32
35. Van Eyck AS, Jordan BF, Gallez B et al (2009) Electron paramagnetic resonance as a tool to evaluate human ovarian tissue reoxygenation after xenografting. Fertil Steril 92:374–381
36. Dolmans MM, Martinez-Madrid B, Gadisseux E et al (2007) Short-term transplantation of isolated human ovarian follicles and cortical tissue into nude mice. Reproduction 134:253–262
37. David A, Van Langendonckt A, Gilliaux S et al (2012) Effect of cryopreservation and transplantation on the expression of kit ligand and anti-Müllerian hormone in human ovarian tissue. Hum Reprod 27:1088–1095
38. Labied S, Delforge Y, Munaut C et al (2013) Isoform 111 of vascular endothelial growth factor (VEGF111) improves angiogenesis of ovarian tissue xenotransplantation. Transplantation 95:426–433
39. Dath C, Dethy A, Van Langendonckt A et al (2011) Endothelial cells are essential for ovarian stromal tissue restructuring after xenotransplantation of isolated ovarian stromal cells. Hum Reprod 26:1431–1439

Chapter 7
Heterotopic Ovarian Tissue Transplantation

Michelle Soares, Marie-Madeleine Dolmans, and Jacques Donnez

Abstract Restoration of ovarian function has been consistently observed after transplantation of ovarian tissue to heterotopic sites, and recent reports now confirm that ovarian function following heterotopic transplantation can last more than 7 years, depending on the initial ovarian reserve. The possibility of long-term restoration of ovarian function, combined with the advantage of a less invasive and more cost-efficient procedure (especially when considering repeated transplantations), makes heterotopic transplantation the technique of choice when the main goal of grafting is restoration of endocrine function.

Although follicle development, oocyte retrieval and fertilization, and embryo development have been demonstrated after heterotopic transplantation of frozen-thawed ovarian tissue to various heterotopic sites, oocyte quality, and hence embryo quality, appear to be compromised. This is probably attributable to the nonoptimal environment for follicular development. Teams who have simultaneously grafted ovarian tissue to orthotopic as well as heterotopic sites report superior results with orthotopic sites. Therefore, when fertility restoration is the goal, there is no doubt that orthotopic sites in the pelvic cavity (ovarian medulla or pelvic peritoneum), although more invasive, are much more effective, as evidenced by the number of live births.

Moreover, grafting of ovarian tissue to a subperitoneal pocket in the abdominal wall could potentially be an option in case of severe pelvic adhesions that preclude pelvic surgery, or in addition to grafting to orthotopic sites, and should be investigated further.

Keywords Heterotopic • Ovarian tissue transplantation • Grafting site

---

M. Soares
Pôle de Recherche en Gynécologie, Institut Expérimental et Clinique, Université Catholique de Louvain, Avenue Mounier 52, bte B1.52.02, 1200 Brussels, Belgium

M.-M. Dolmans (✉)
Pôle de Recherche en Gynécologie, Institut Expérimental et Clinique, Université Catholique de Louvain, Avenue Mounier 52, bte B1.52.02, 1200 Brussels, Belgium

Département de Gynécologie, Cliniques Universitaires Saint-Luc, Brussels, Belgium
e-mail: marie-madeleine.dolmans@uclouvain.be

J. Donnez
Société de Recherche pour l'Infertilité, Brussels, Belgium

N. Suzuki, J. Donnez (eds.), *Gonadal Tissue Cryopreservation in Fertility Preservation*, DOI 10.1007/978-4-431-55963-4_7

7.1 Introduction

Ovarian tissue transplantation has a long history, dating back to 1895, when the first graft was performed by Robert Morris. However, due to the lack of good clinical indications, interest in human ovarian tissue grafting gradually waned until the development of new technologies for assisted reproduction and cryopreservation. Almost 100 years after the first transplant, interest in human ovarian tissue transplantation was once again reignited in 1994, when Gosden et al. demonstrated fertility restoration after frozen-thawed ovarian tissue transplantation in sheep [1]. Since then, ovarian tissue cryopreservation and transplantation has become a key topic in reproductive medicine.

Today, cryopreservation of ovarian tissue is gaining ground as an established fertility preservation technique. It is the only currently available option for prepubescent girls and women with cancer who cannot delay the start of cancer treatment, and can be combined with immature oocyte retrieval followed by in vitro maturation.

Reimplantation of cryopreserved ovarian tissue has become clinically feasible and is practiced in a number of centers worldwide. Since the first live birth following frozen-thawed ovarian tissue transplantation in a woman with Hodgkin's lymphoma in 2004 [2], 60 more live births ([3], + see chapter by J. Donnez in the present book) have been reported in the literature to date, showing that this technique should no longer be considered experimental.

Ovarian tissue has been transplanted back to orthotopic as well as heterotopic sites, and the choice of transplantation site constitutes an essential factor in future graft viability and oocyte quality and competence. Before proceeding any further, it is important to clearly define what is meant by orthotopic and heterotopic, as the use of different terminology can lead to misunderstandings.

Strictly speaking, orthotopic ovarian tissue transplantation implies grafting of ovarian cortical strips to their natural site, namely the remaining ovary. However, grafting of this tissue to pelvic sites in general, including the pelvic peritoneum and broad ligaments where environmental conditions are very close to natural, is also widely considered to be orthotopic [4]. While restoration of endocrine function and fertility have been demonstrated following orthotopic transplantation, efficacy and success rates are still not really known because the denominator is unknown. In a recently published report (5) combining results from 5 fertility centers [5–8], the pregnancy rate (based on the number of women who conceived) following orthotopic transplantation was 29 % (32 out of 111).

Heterotopic sites, namely sites that have nothing to do with the natural localization or environment of the ovary, like the forearm (subcutaneous (SC)), abdominal wall (SC, intramuscular (IM), just below the fascia), and chest wall (pectoralis muscle), have also been used for grafting of ovarian cortical strips and are associated with restoration of ovarian function and follicular development with oocyte retrieval. Nevertheless, just one (twin) live birth has been reported to date [9].

After a general overview of the history of ovarian tissue grafting, this chapter will address the specifics of heterotopic transplantation, including different grafting sites, advantages and limitations, experimental and clinical results, and factors affecting graft function after transplantation.

7.2 History of Ovarian Tissue Transplantation

Ovarian tissue grafting has a long history, beginning with a small account that appeared in the thesis of Paul Bert in 1863 [10, 11]. The initially disappointing results apparently dulled interest for the next 30 years. These early studies often used implants of ovarian tissue slices, showing their capacity to survive following rapid revascularization. Early studies on human ovarian tissue transplantation for fertility restoration or as treatment for menopausal symptoms described menstrual cyclicity, pregnancies, and even deliveries after grafting, as reported in a review by Nugent et al. [10]. Some also claimed success with ovarian tissue allografts, believing the ovary to have a certain degree of immunological privilege. However, current knowledge of immunology indicates that these claims were somewhat overstated, and we now know that immunosuppressive therapies are essential if ovarian allografts are to survive. Although the scientific validity of this early work is questionable, the concept of ovarian implants remains attractive.

In humans, the first ovarian implants were reported by Robert Morris in a woman suffering from ovarian failure as far back as 1895 [12]. The patient reportedly became pregnant, but it ended in spontaneous miscarriage. Other similar transplants were described in the years that followed, with variable outcomes.

Orthotopic transplantation to the broad ligament was then the procedure of choice to obtain pregnancy due to its simplicity. Nonetheless, it proved disappointing from a fertility point of view, and ovarian transposition (including the vascular pedicle) to the uterine cavity [13] or uterine horn [14] appeared to yield better results.

As potential treatment for menopausal symptoms, the graft site was not an issue, and many heterotopic sites were tested: the rectus muscle, skin of the abdomen, omentum, cervix, and saphenous vein [10]. Cycles of normal length could be restored by grafting to these heterotopic locations, as long as a satisfactory blood supply was available, the only exception being portal circulation. Indeed, in this site, hepatic clearance of steroid hormones reduces negative feedback on gonadotropin secretion, causing graft hyperstimulation. With the advent of high-resolution ultrasound and in vitro fertilization (IVF) techniques, heterotopic ovarian transplantation began to be considered a potential option for fertility preservation, either by reimplanting slices of frozen-thawed tissue or by grafting fresh tissue to sites outside the radiation field. In 1987, Le Porrier et al. heterotopically transplanted the ovary of a patient with subdiaphragmatic Hodgkin's disease to the SC tissue of the arm [15]. This resulted in regular menstrual cycles, with observable cyclic changes to the circumference of the arm. A year after surgery, a secondary oocyte was recovered.

Advances made in the field of cryobiology over these last 30 years now allow successful cryopreservation techniques for human ovarian tissue and led to the introduction of ovarian tissue freezing as an option to preserve female fertility in the late 1990s.

Transplantation of cryopreserved ovarian tissue has been successfully performed in different animal models (rodents, rabbits, sheep, and marmoset monkeys [1, 16, 17]). In 2000, the first case of successful orthotopic autotransplantation of frozen-thawed ovarian tissue was reported in humans [18]. Ovarian tissue was transplanted to peritoneal pockets in the pelvic peritoneum of a woman who had previously undergone bilateral oophorectomy, resulting in follicle development and ovulation 15 weeks later, after gonadotropin administration. The following year, Callejo et al. described the same after autografting frozen-thawed tissue to a heterotopic site (rectus muscle of the abdomen) [19]. The first human live birth issuing from the orthotopic technique was reported in 2004 [2] and, since then, at least 42 more live births have been achieved by several centers worldwide after orthotopic transplantation (see chapter on orthotopic transplantation). On the other hand, just one twin delivery has been documented after grafting to a subperitoneal pocket in the abdominal wall, while no pregnancies have been obtained with SC or IM sites.

7.3 Optimal Heterotopic Site

7.3.1 Animal Studies

A number of experiments conducted in animal models after ovarian tissue autografting or xenografting have evaluated follicle development potential in various heterotopic sites, allowing comparison with orthotopic sites.

Different studies in rodents show the kidney capsule or ovarian bursa to have an advantage over SC or intraperitoneal (IP) locations [20–22]. Using a xenografting model, Israely et al. showed better follicle preservation and less tissue damage in rat ovaries transplanted to an IM site in mice compared to an SC site. In a xenotransplantation study of human ovarian tissue to nude mice, four grafting sites (peritoneum, ovarian bursa, SC, and IM) were found to equally support early follicular growth and preserve some quiescent follicles, although a lower degree of fibrosis was observed in the IM site [23]. In another study comparing the kidney capsule to the back muscle as a grafting site in mice, Soleimani et al. reported better follicle survival in grafts from the back muscle.

Since the primary aim of ovarian tissue transplantation is fertility restoration, evaluation of oocyte quality and competence and normal embryo development are important prerequisites for human application. Different studies to date have shown that oocytes collected from grafted ovarian tissue, depending on graft site, exhibited lower embryo development potential than controls [24–27]. Subcutaneously grafted ovaries in mice had a lower oocyte yield compared to ovaries placed in the kidney capsule or ovarian bursa, while more embryos developed from oocytes retrieved from tissue grafted to the ovarian bursa, even though implantation rates did not differ [27]. Another study demonstrated that oocytes recovered and further matured in vitro after xenografting of human ovarian tissue subcutaneously to SCID mice showed aberrant microtubule organization and chromatin patterns.

Several reports of live young obtained after IVF of oocytes retrieved from SC [27, 28] and IM [29] grafts in mice have been published. In monkeys, the only live birth derived from an SC graft (fresh tissue) occurred in an animal whose resulting embryos were transferred to a gestational surrogate [30]. Other grafting sites, like the pouch of Douglas, omentum, retroperitoneal iliac fossa, mesosalpinx, uterine serosa, and pelvic wall, have also been tested in primates [31, 32]. One of these studies revealed that an omental location was associated with better follicle survival and development than the abdominal wall or pouch of Douglas [31].

7.4 Clinical Experience of Heterotopic Ovarian Tissue Transplantation in Humans

In humans, different heterotopic sites have been investigated since the first graft in 1895. These include the forearm [33, 34], SC tissue of the abdomen [19, 35], breast tissue [36], rectus muscle [36–38], and the anterior wall of the abdomen, just beneath the peritoneum [9, 39, 40].

Clinical studies on heterotopic autotransplantation of cryopreserved ovarian tissue are still limited and summarized in Table 7.1. In 2001, Callejo et al. evaluated the long-term function of fresh (three patients) and frozen (one patient) ovarian tissue grafted subcutaneously to the arm or rectus muscle of the abdomen [19]. Ovarian activity resumed 3–4 months after the procedure in three of the four patients. However, as the patients were premenopausal (46–49 years) at the time of ovarian tissue cryopreservation, no conclusions could be drawn.

In the same year, Oktay et al. described SC fresh ovarian tissue transplantation to the forearm in a 35-year-old patient with stage III squamous cell carcinoma of the cervix and a 37-year-old patient with recurrent benign serous ovarian cysts [33]. Ovarian function resumed 10 weeks and 5 months after transplantation respectively. One MII oocyte obtained after ovarian stimulation in patient 1 failed to fertilize. Graft function lasted more than 21 months in both cases.

These early studies confirmed that simple ovarian grafts, either fresh or cryopreserved, could form functional tissue when grafted to heterotopic sites in women, without any vascular anastomosis.

Later, Kim et al. reported transplantation of cryopreserved ovarian tissue to the rectus muscle (abdominal site, technique shown in Fig. 7.1) and pectoralis muscle (breast site) in a 37-year-old patient cured of squamous cell carcinoma of the cervix

Table 7.1 Heterotopic transplantation of cryopreserved ovarian tissue

Reference/group	Age before freezing	Chemotherapy before freezing	Indication	Graft site (1st and 2nd transplants)	Grafted strips (size and number per transplant)	Time to recovery of ovarian function: 1st/2nd transplant	Life-span of the graft (months): 1st/2nd transplant	Outcome from heterotopic site
Callejo et al. [19]	47	No	Uterine leiomyoma	Rectus abdominis muscle	Size: 2–3 mm^3 Pcs: 40–45	3–4 months	5–6	↑ E2, FD after stimulation (follicle of 20 mm)
Kim et al. ([36], [65])	37	No	Cervical cancer	1st: A (between rectus muscle and sheath) + B (between breast tissue and pectoralis muscle)	Size: 5 × 5 × 1–2 mm	14 weeks	4/14	↑ E2, ↓ FSH
				2nd: A (rectus muscle)	Pcs: 1st: 20 (B) + 20 (A) 2nd: 20 (A)			FD (follicle of 11–16 mm) only in A site, ovulation
	NA	No	Cervical cancer	A (rectus muscle)	NA	3–5 months/ 2–4 months	NA	Disease relapse, patient expired 5 months after the graft
	28	No	Cervical cancer	1st and 2nd: A (rectus muscle)	Size: 5 × 5 × 1–2 mm Pcs: 1st: 9 2nd: 8		6/84	↑ E2, ↓ FSH, FD *3 IVF cycles: 6 oocytes (1 GV, 4 MI, 1 MII) -> 4 embryos (6-cell, 3-cell, 2-cell, and pronuclear stage*
	29	No	Breast cancer	1st and 2nd: A (rectus muscle)	Size: 5× 5× 1–2 mm Pcs: 1st: 11 2nd: 8		5/9	All embryos cryopreserved
	30	No	Hodgkin's lymphoma	1st and 2nd: A (rectus muscle)	Size: 5 × 5 × 1–2 mm Pcs: 1st: 10 2nd: 8		9/→	↑ E2, ↓ FSH, FD

Oktay et al. ([41], [42], [43])	30	No	Breast cancer	A (SC)	Size: 5 × 5 × 1–15 × 5 × 2 mm Pcs: 15	3 months	62→	FD after gonadotrophin stimulation 20 oocytes -> 8 IVF-ICSI ->2 embryos: one 4-cell (transferred) + one aneuploidic
	28	Yes	Hodgkin's lymphoma	A (SC)	Left ovary in pieces	2 months	42→	FD, ovulation 1 MII oocyte recovered → no fertilization N.B. Spontaneous pregnancy with 3 LB after transplantation
Wolner-Hanssen et al. [34]	30	No	Pure red cell aplasia + BMT	Forearm (SC)	Size: 1–2 × 1–2 × 0.5–1 mm Pcs: 10	18 weeks	NA	FD (follicles of 12.6 mm and 6.7 mm) after local gonadotrophin stimulation
Rosendahl et al. [9] and Schmidt et al. [44]	32	No	Hodgkin	1st: O 2nd: O + A (SP)	Size: 5 × 5 × 1 mm Pcs: 1st: 4 (O) 2nd: 8 (O) + 4 (A)	8/12 weeks	45/23	2 IVF cycles: no oocyte from A
	28	Yes	Hodgkin's relapse	1st: O + P + A (SP) 2nd: O + A (SP)	Size: 5 × 5 × 1 mm Pcs: 1st: 4 (O) + 4 (P) + 4 (A) 2nd: 4 (0) + 4 (A)	19 weeks/1st still functioning	54→/12→	9 IVF cycles: I empty zona + 2 MII oocytes retrieved -> 2 embryos -> 1 biochemical pregnancy
	25	Yes	Hodgkin's relapse	1st: O + P + A (SP) 2nd: O + A (SP)	Size: 5 × 5 × 1 mm Pcs: 1st: 3 (O) + 4 (A) + 5 (P) 2nd: 5 (O) + 1 (A)	18/16 weeks	26/39→	12 IVF cycles: no oocyte from A
	19	No	Paroxymsal nocturnal hemoglobinuria (PNH)	O + A (SP)	Size: 5 × 5 × 1 mm Pcs: 7 (O) + 5 (A)	15 weeks	18→	3 IVF cycles: I empty zona + 3 MII oocytes retrieved -> 1 embryo -> no pregnancy
	25	No	Aplastic anemia	O + A (SP)	Size: 5 × 5 × 1 mm Pcs: 5 (O) + 2 (A)	26 weeks	13 →	3 IVF cycles: I irregular +1 MII oocyte retrieved -> failed to fertilize

(continued)

Table 7.1 (continued)

Reference/group	Age before freezing	Chemotherapy before freezing	Indication	Graft site (1st and 2nd transplants)	Grafted strips (size and number per transplant)	Time to recovery of ovarian function: 1st/2nd transplant	Life-span of the graft (months): 1st/2nd transplant	Outcome from heterotopic site
Demeestere et al. [35], [45]	24	Yes	Hodgkin's	1st: O + P (2 step) + A (SC)	Size: 5 × 5 × 2 mm	3 months	~12/NA	↑ E2, ↓ FSH, FD at all sites
				2nd: O + P (2 step)+ A (SC)	Pcs:			Follicles at A site reached a max of 13 mm
					1st: 3 (O) + 9 (P) + 6 (A)			N.B. LB from spontaneous ovulation at O site
					2nd: 2 (O) + 2 (A)			
Stern et al. [39], [40], 2014 [46]	17	Yes	Non-Hodgkin's lymphoma	1st: O + P + A (SP)	Size: 4 × 2 × 1 mm	8.5/3 months	17/NA	FD at all 3 graft sites
				2nd: O + P + A (SP)	Pcs: 80 mm^3			9 IVF cycles: at least 1 oocytes from A site
	21	No	Granulosa cell tumor	1st: P + A (SP)	Size: 4 × 2 × 1 mm	4.5 months	24/NA	↑ E2, ↓ FSH
				2nd: A (SP)	Pcs:			*1st graft*: Multiple mild stimulation cycles -> 3 oocytes -> 2 embryos -> no pregnancy
					1st: 30 (P) + 30 (A)			FD seen at Lps 2 years after Tx
					2nd: 60 (A)			*2nd graft:* Two IVF cycles: 2 MII oocytes from A -> 8-cell and 5-cell embryo -> twin delivery
								N.B. Disease recurrence observed at C-section

"→" in life span column = still ongoing at the time of submission
NA not available
In graft site column: *A* anterior abdominal wall, *SC* subcutaneous, *SP* subperitoneal, *B* breast, *O* ovary, *P* pelvic peritoneum
FD follicle development, *E2* estradiol, *GV* germinal vesicle, *Pcs* pieces, *LB* live birth

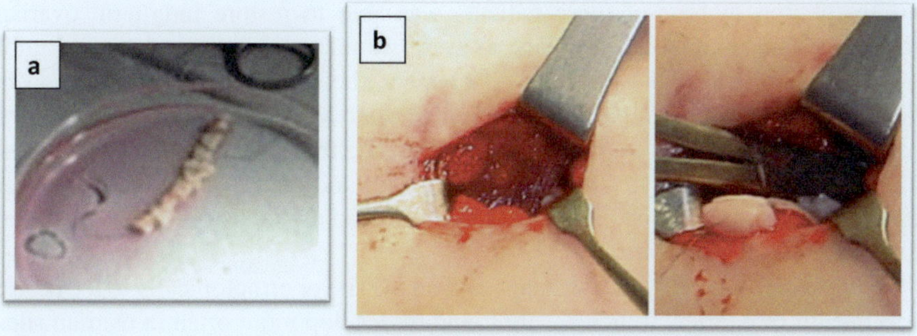

Fig. 7.1 Process of transplantation of frozen-thawed ovarian tissue to a heterotopic site in the abdominal wall. (**a**) Thin ovarian cortex is threaded onto a 3-0 Vicryl suture and (**b**) transplanted between the rectus muscle and its sheath through a small skin incision (2 cm) (pictures taken from **a** Kim et al. [37] and **b** Kim et al. [38]

[36]. Restoration of ovarian function was detected 14 weeks after transplantation, but unfortunately activity ceased around 28 weeks after transplantation, as evidenced by high follicle-stimulating hormone (FSH) and very low estradiol levels.

Around the same time, Oktay et al. reported a case of embryo development from an oocyte retrieved after implantation of frozen-thawed ovarian tissue beneath the skin of the abdomen in a woman with breast cancer. After eight retrieval attempts, just 8 of the 20 oocytes obtained were suitable for IVF and only one fertilized to give a four-cell embryo, but no pregnancy was achieved after transplantation. This study indicated that ovarian follicles with viable and functional oocytes can develop in frozen-thawed ovarian tissue transplanted to a heterotopic site, but also suggested that oocyte quality may be compromised in this heterotopic location. Although freezing and thawing procedures and initial ischemia could be partially responsible for this, these poor results are also attributable to suboptimal environmental factors for follicle development, like pressure, temperature, and paracrine factors in heterotopic sites, compared to those in the peritoneal cavity.

In 2005, Wolner-Hanssen et al. [34] reported the development of two follicles after transplantation of thawed ovarian tissue to the forearm. However, these follicles reached a maximum diameter of only 12.6 mm and 6.7 mm respectively, and the life span of the tissue was around 7 months.

More recently, Kim et al. published their 8-year [37] and subsequently 10-year experience in heterotopic transplantation of ovarian tissue in cancer patients, evaluating long-term graft function and fertility restoration ([38]). Between 2001 and 2011, thawed ovarian tissue was transplanted to the space between the rectus muscle and fascia in the abdomen of five cancer survivors (three with cervical cancer, one with breast cancer, and one with Hodgkin's lymphoma) aged between 28 and 35 years. Restoration of ovarian function was observed in all five patients 12–20 weeks after transplantation, as evidenced by the decrease in FSH levels to less than 20 mIU/ml. Graft function lasted only 3–5 months, but a second transplantation in four of these patients was able to restore long-term ovarian function (9–84 months). These patients were stimulated with gonadotropins until a dominant follicle of 14–16 mm was obtained, before oocyte retrieval for IVF. Seven oocytes (two germinal vesicles, four MI, one MII) were recovered from two patients. The MI oocytes were matured in vitro, and three of them developed to full maturity. Four MII oocytes were then fertilized, and the resulting embryos after 2–3 days of culture (six-cell, three-cell, two-cell, and pronuclear stage) were frozen for transfer to a surrogate.

When ovarian tissue was transplanted to an SC site or orthotopically to the pelvic peritoneum or ovaries, follicles were found to develop more often in ovarian sites than in peritoneal or SC sites [35, 45]. Furthermore, follicle development was limited in heterotopic sites (<15 mm), and oocyte recovery and fertilization rates obtained from SC sites were low [35].

In 2006, a Danish group reported a biochemical pregnancy resulting from transfer of a four-cell embryo obtained after intracytoplasmic sperm injection, following retrieval of an MII oocyte from tissue grafted to a midline subperitoneal pocket on the lower abdominal wall [9]. Two months later, a second MII oocyte was recovered and fertilized, and a five-cell embryo was transferred, but no pregnancy was achieved. In their series of 12 autotransplantations of cryopreserved ovarian tissue published in 2011 [44], ovarian tissue was grafted to this same heterotopic site in five patients, in addition to other orthotopic sites (remaining ovary and pelvic peritoneum). After stimulation and IVF, tissue grafted to the subperitoneal pocket was shown to yield mature oocytes after IVF in three patients, but no pregnancy was reported from this site, compared to two live births and a higher number of embryos obtained from orthotopic locations.

A second biochemical pregnancy following ovarian grafting to this same site was reported by Stern et al. in 2011. Recently, the same group published their first pregnancy and live birth (twins) [39, 46] following heterotopic grafting of frozen-thawed ovarian tissue. However, in this case, the tissue was laparoscopically transplanted to a subperitoneal area of the anterior abdominal peritoneum (along with the lateral pelvic peritoneum) in a patient who had previously undergone bilateral oophorectomy for a granulosa cell tumor. This site, just below the peritoneum, was considered heterotopic by this team. However, laparoscopic visualization of the grafts confirms the presence of cystic follicular structures protruding into the peritoneal cavity (Fig. 7.2), very similar to what is observed after orthotopic grafting of tissue to the pelvic peritoneum (orthotopic site). It is therefore questionable whether this graft can truly be considered heterotopic.

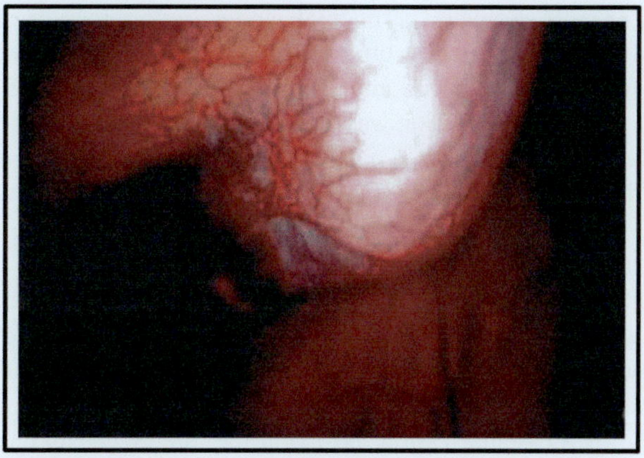

Fig. 7.2 Laparoscopic view of the abdominal wall ovarian tissue graft two years after transplantation, showing cystic follicular structures protruding into the peritoneal cavity (picture from Stern et al. [39])

7.5 Factors Influencing Graft Function After Transplantation

The choice of grafting site is an important factor when considering future graft viability and subsequent follicle development and oocyte competence. Apart from graft site (environment), factors influencing graft function after heterotopic transplantation are partially the same as for orthotopic transplantation. They include the following:

7.5.1 Clinical Considerations

The life span of an ovarian graft is influenced by various clinical factors, like the number and size of grafted tissue and the surgical technique used. However, the most important among them is follicle density in the cryopreserved tissue, which depends on the age of the patient at the time of ovarian tissue cryopreservation and any prior gonadotoxic treatment she may have undergone. Previous gonadotoxic treatment could decrease the follicular pool, but also interfere with the revascularization process after grafting, as chemotherapy causes injury to blood vessels and cortical fibrosis [47].

7.5.2 Vascularization

Since ovarian tissue grafting is an avascular procedure, survival of the transplant is hugely dependent on the revascularization process. Indeed, ischemic injury occurring immediately after transplantation is associated with massive initial follicle loss

[48, 49]. Some experimental studies report loss of at least 25 % of primordial follicles [50], while others put the figure as high as 50–65 % of the primordial follicle pool [48, 51] and even >90 % in one study [25].

In mice, perfusion was observed in autografts 3 days after grafting [52]. A study analyzing angiogenic events following rat ovary transplantation to nude mice by dynamic contrast-enhanced magnetic resonance imaging (MRI) detected functional vessels in grafts from day 7 onward [53]. In humans, neovascularization was observed 3 days after transplantation to chick chorioallantoic membrane [54]. Another study using electron paramagnetic resonance (EPR) oximetry showed a hypoxic period before day 5 after xenotransplantation of human ovarian tissue, followed by progressive reoxygenation during the subsequent 5 days [55]. The same group demonstrated that host and graft vessels contributed sequentially to graft revascularization; host (murine) angiogenesis initiated reperfusion from day 5, but by day 10, human angiogenesis was found to participate in graft revascularization [56].

Prevention of ischemic tissue damage, which remains one of the main limitations of ovarian cortical strip use, is therefore essential to reduce follicle loss.

7.5.3 Addition of Exogenous Factors

Addition of exogenous factors has also been investigated, with the aim of shortening the ischemic period following transplantation and increasing the viability and reproductive potential of grafts.

7.5.3.1 Growth and Angiogenic Factors

Various angiogenic and growth factors known to play a role in revascularization processes have been tested in xenotransplantation models. Sphingosine-1-phosphate (S1P) was shown to promote neoangiogenesis in ovarian transplants and reduce ischemia-reperfusion injury in the days following transplantation in a mouse xenograft model [57]. Erythropoietin was found to improve early follicle morphology, stromal cell density, and blood vessel density [58, 59]. Although earlier studies with vascular endothelial growth factor (VEGF) failed to demonstrate any positive effect on graft function [24], encapsulation of ovarian tissue in a collagen matrix in the presence of VEGF-165 before grafting was recently shown to have a positive impact on functional blood vessel recruitment [60]. Another study demonstrated that administration of VEGF and basic fibroblast growth factor (bFGF), especially combined, was found to trigger angiogenesis, reduce apoptosis and fibrosis, and increase survival of human ovarian tissue transplanted to rabbits [61]. Use of growth factors to improve ovarian tissue survival after grafting has progressed beyond the preclinical stage. One group reported a live birth after impregnation of frozen-thawed ovarian cortex with platelet-rich plasma and orthotopic reimplantation [62].

The gonadotropins, luteinizing hormone (LH) and FSH, are follicle survival factors with possible antiapoptotic action and are known to upregulate angiogenic factors like VEGF. Gonadotropin administration for a few days increases the number of growing follicles in grafts when initiated 2–4 days before transplantation [20, 63]. However, no effect is observed on follicle populations when started immediately after grafting [52].

7.5.3.2 Antioxidants

Reactive oxygen species (ROS) produced during the ischemia-reperfusion period are widely implicated in causing damage to cells and massive activation of primary follicles. Endogenous antioxidant molecules are produced to neutralize these free oxygen radicals, but are rapidly overwhelmed. Nugent et al. [52] reported an improvement in follicle survival rates after local vitamin E injection before grafting, but these findings were not corroborated by others [64, 65]. Abir et al. [65] compared incubation of ovarian tissue with VEGF-A and vitamin E before transplantation, and treatment of host mice with vitamin E and gonadotropins before and after grafting, with control groups. Although apoptosis was higher in the non-treated group, no difference was found in the number of total and atretic follicles between the groups.

Melatonin and oxytetracycline, two more antioxidants, were shown to decrease graft necrosis when administered locally during intraperitoneal ovarian tissue grafting in rats [66]. The efficacy of ascorbic acid was also tested on bovine ovarian cortex deprived of a blood supply [67]. Primordial follicles were found to be less sensitive to ischemic injury than stromal cells, and incubating the tissue in ascorbic acid reduced apoptosis for up to 24 hours.

A recent study evaluating the impact of adding N-acetylcysteine (NAC) to freeze/thawing solutions showed reduced ROS production and better preservation of morphological characteristics, proliferation, and DNA integrity of ovarian tissue with NAC [68].

Even if these results are encouraging, further studies are required to establish the positive effects of such growth factors and antioxidants on follicle development and fertility restoration, and to precisely define the cytokines that may be of significant clinical benefit in terms of ovarian grafting efficiency.

7.6 Advantages and Disadvantages of Heterotopic Ovarian Transplantation

The advantages and disadvantages of heterotopic ovarian transplantation are summarized in Table 7.2. In theory, the optimal grafting site should have a rich blood supply, mimic the environmental conditions of the ovary in the peritoneum, and offer easy access for both implantation and oocyte recovery.

Transplantation to a heterotopic site is a relatively simple and minimally invasive procedure. It can also be performed in patients with severe pelvic adhesions and those in whom orthotopic transplantation is precluded. These aspects, along with easy accessibility for follicle monitoring and oocyte retrieval (in more superficial sites), are its major advantages compared to orthotopic transplantation. Another benefit of this technique is the ability to closely monitor the graft for possible recurrence of malignancy. Heterotopic sites also allow grafting of larger amounts of tissue.

However, unlike orthotopic transplantation, heterotopic transplantation does not allow natural conception, and patients are obliged to undergo IVF in order to achieve pregnancy. Moreover, obtaining healthy and competent oocytes from these grafts for IVF still remains a considerable challenge. Although restoration of ovarian activity and oocyte retrieval after grafting to heterotopic sites have been confirmed by several teams, follicular growth appears to be compromised, and recovered oocytes are mostly of inferior quality. This is probably due to the suboptimal environment of heterotopic sites. Indeed, environmental conditions in most heterotopic locations (pressure, temperature, cytokines, space for follicular

Table 7.2 Advantages and disadvantages of heterotopic ovarian tissue transplantation

	Heterotopic sites (e.g. SC)	Orthotopic sites (ovary and pelvic peritoneum)
Advantages	Simple and less invasive transplantation procedure	Possibility of natural pregnancy
	Easy access for follicle monitoring and oocyte recovery	Favorable environment for follicular development
	No limit to the number of grafted fragments	Restoration of fertility demonstrated with follicle development and oocyte quality superior to heterotopic sites
	Possibility to closely monitor for recurrence of malignancy in the graft	
Disadvantages	IVF procedure required	Invasive transplantation procedure requiring general anesthesia
	Probable suboptimal environmental conditions for oocyte development	For the ovarian site, number of grafted fragments limited by ovarian size
	Cosmetic issues	
	Restoration of fertility not demonstrated	

growth, angiogenic and hormonal factors ([37, 38]) are not equivalent to those in an orthotopic site in the pelvis.

7.7 Conclusion: The Future of Heterotopic Ovarian Tissue Transplantation

It is important to choose well vascularized grafting sites, as the major cause of follicle loss after ovarian transplantation is ischemic injury. Concerning restoration of ovarian function, this has been consistently observed after transplantation of ovarian tissue to heterotopic sites. Recent reports confirm that ovarian function following heterotopic transplantation can last more than 7 years, depending on the initial ovarian reserve [38]. The possibility of long-term restoration of ovarian function, combined with the advantage of a less invasive and more cost-efficient procedure (especially when considering repeated transplantations), makes heterotopic transplantation the technique of choice when the main goal of grafting is restoration of endocrine function.

Although follicular development, oocyte retrieval and fertilization, and embryo development have been confirmed after heterotopic transplantation of frozen-thawed ovarian tissue to various heterotopic sites, oocyte quality, and hence embryo quality, appear to be compromised [9, 36, 37, 38]. Teams who have simultaneously grafted ovarian tissue to orthotopic as well as heterotopic sites report superior results with orthotopic sites [35, 44]. Alterations in oocyte quality described in heterotopic sites are probably attributable to the nonoptimal environment for follicular development. Therefore, when fertility restoration is the goal, there is no doubt that orthotopic sites in the pelvic cavity (ovarian medulla or pelvic peritoneum), although more invasive, are much more effective, as evidenced by the number of live births.

Moreover, grafting of ovarian tissue to a subperitoneal pocket in the abdominal wall could also potentially be an option in case of severe pelvic adhesions that preclude pelvic surgery, or in addition to grafting to orthotopic sites, and should be investigated further.

References

1. Gosden RG, Baird DT, Wade JC, Webb R (1994) Restoration of fertility to oophorectomized sheep by ovarian autografts stored at -196 degrees C. Hum Reprod 9(4):597–603
2. Donnez J, Dolmans MM, Demylle D, Jadoul P, Pirard C, Squifflet J et al (2004) Livebirth after orthotopic transplantation of cryopreserved ovarian tissue. Lancet 364(9443):1405–1410
3. Donnez J, Dolmans MM (2015) Ovarian cortex transplantation: 60 reported live births brings the success and worldwide expansion of the technique towards routine clinical practice. J Assist Reprod Genet 32:1167–1170

4. Donnez J, Dolmans MM, Diaz C, Pellicer A (2015) Ovarian cortex transplantation: time to move on from experimental studies to open clinical application. Fertil Steril 104(5):1097–1098
5. Practice Committee of American Society for Reproductive Medicine (2014) Ovarian tissue cryopreservation: a committee opinion. Fertil Steril 101(5):1237–43
6. Macklon KT, Jensen AK, Loft A, Ernst E, Andersen CY (2014) Treatment history and outcome of 24 deliveries worldwide after autotransplantation of cryopreserved ovarian tissue, including two new Danish deliveries years after autotransplantation. J Assist Reprod Genet 31 (11):1557–1564
7. Donnez J, Dolmans MM, Pellicer A, Diaz-Garcia C, Sanchez Serrano M, Schmidt KT et al (2013) Restoration of ovarian activity and pregnancy after transplantation of cryopreserved ovarian tissue: a review of 60 cases of reimplantation. Fertil Steril 99 (6):1503–1513
8. Dittrich R, Hackl J, Lotz L, Hoffmann I, Beckmann MW (2015) Pregnancies and live births after 20 transplantations of cryopreserved ovarian tissue in a single center. Fertil Steril 103 (2):462–468
9. Rosendahl M, Loft A, Byskov AG, Ziebe S, Schmidt KT, Andersen AN et al (2006) Biochemical pregnancy after fertilization of an oocyte aspirated from a heterotopic autotransplant of cryopreserved ovarian tissue: case report. Hum Reprod 21(8):2006–2009
10. Nugent D, Meirow D, Brook PF, Aubard Y, Gosden RG (1997) Transplantation in reproductive medicine: previous experience, present knowledge and future prospects. Hum Reprod Update 3(3):267–280
11. Gosden RG (2008) Ovary and uterus transplantation. Reproduction 136(6):671–680
12. Morris RT (1895) The ovarian graft. N Y Med J 62:436
13. Dudley PA (1900) A further report on ovarian implantation. Cong Int Med CR Sect Gyne xv:387–388
14. Estes WL (1909) A method of implanting ovarian tissue in order to maintain ovarian function. Pennsylv Med J 13:610–613
15. Leporrier M, von Theobald P, Roffe JL, Muller G (1987) A new technique to protect ovarian function before pelvic irradiation. Heterotopic ovarian autotransplantation. Cancer 60 (9):2201–2204
16. Candy CJ, Wood MJ, Whittingham DG (1995) Follicular development in cryopreserved marmoset ovarian tissue after transplantation. Hum Reprod 10(9):2334–2338
17. Candy CJ, Wood MJ, Whittingham DG (2000) Restoration of a normal reproductive lifespan after grafting of cryopreserved mouse ovaries. Hum Reprod 15(6):1300–1304
18. Oktay K, Karlikaya G (2000) Ovarian function after transplantation of frozen, banked autologous ovarian tissue. N Engl J Med 342(25):1919
19. Callejo J, Salvador C, Miralles A, Vilaseca S, Lailla JM, Balasch J (2001) Long-term ovarian function evaluation after autografting by implantation with fresh and frozen-thawed human ovarian tissue. J Clin Endocrinol Metab 86(9):4489–4494
20. Imthurn B, Cox SL, Jenkin G, Trounson AO, Shaw JM (2000) Gonadotrophin administration can benefit ovarian tissue grafted to the body wall: implications for human ovarian grafting. Mol Cell Endocrinol 163(1–2):141–146
21. Callejo J, Vilaseca S, Ordi J, Cabre S, Lailla JM, Balasch J (2002) Heterotopic ovarian transplantation without vascular pedicle in syngeneic Lewis rats: long-term evaluation of effects on ovarian structure and function. Fertil Steril 77(2):396–402
22. Risvanli A, Timurkan H, Akpolat N, Gulacti I, Ulakoglu E (2006) A study of ovarian autotransplantation without vascular a pedicle in rats. J Assist Reprod Genet 23 (11–12):401–406
23. Dath C, Van Eyck AS, Dolmans MM, Romeu L, Delle Vigne L, Donnez J et al (2010) Xenotransplantation of human ovarian tissue to nude mice: comparison between four grafting sites. Hum Reprod 25(7):1734–1743
24. Demeestere I, Simon P, Emiliani S, Delbaere A, Englert Y (2009) Orthotopic and heterotopic ovarian tissue transplantation. Hum Reprod Update 15(6):649–665

25. Aubard Y, Piver P, Cogni Y, Fermeaux V, Poulin N, Driancourt MA (1999) Orthotopic and heterotopic autografts of frozen-thawed ovarian cortex in sheep. Hum Reprod 14 (8):2149–2154
26. Waterhouse T, Cox SL, Snow M, Jenkin G, Shaw J (2004) Offspring produced from heterotopic ovarian allografts in male and female recipient mice. Reproduction 127(6):689–694
27. Yang HY, Cox SL, Jenkin G, Findlay J, Trounson A, Shaw J (2006) Graft site and gonadotrophin stimulation influences the number and quality of oocytes from murine ovarian tissue grafts. Reproduction 131(5):851–859
28. Mitsui A, Yoshizawa M (2007) Successful pregnancy in ovariectomized mice using a combination of heterotopic autotransplantation of ovarian tissues and embryo transfer. Reprod Med Biol 6(2):85–90
29. Soleimani R, Van der Elst J, Heytens E, Van den Broecke R, Gerris J, Dhont M et al (2008) Back muscle as a promising site for ovarian tissue transplantation, an animal model. Hum Reprod 23(3):619–626
30. Lee DM, Yeoman RR, Battaglia DE, Stouffer RL, Zelinski-Wooten MB, Fanton JW et al (2004) Live birth after ovarian tissue transplant. Nature 428(6979):137–138
31. Diaz-Garcia C, Milenkovic M, Groth K, Dahm-Kahler P, Olausson M, Brannstrom M (2011) Ovarian cortex transplantation in the baboon: comparison of four different intra-abdominal transplantation sites. Hum Reprod 26(12):3303–3311
32. Suzuki N, Hashimoto S, Igarashi S, Takae S, Yamanaka M, Yamochi T et al (2012) Assessment of long-term function of heterotopic transplants of vitrified ovarian tissue in cynomolgus monkeys. Hum Reprod 27(8):2420–2429
33. Oktay K, Economos K, Kan M, Rucinski J, Veeck L, Rosenwaks Z (2001) Endocrine function and oocyte retrieval after autologous transplantation of ovarian cortical strips to the forearm. JAMA 286(12):1490–1493
34. Wolner-Hanssen P, Hagglund L, Ploman F, Ramirez A, Manthorpe R, Thuring A (2005) Autotransplantation of cryopreserved ovarian tissue to the right forearm 4(1/2) years after autologous stem cell transplantation. Acta Obstet Gynecol Scand 84(7):695–698
35. Demeestere I, Simon P, Buxant F, Robin V, Fernandez SA, Centner J et al (2006) Ovarian function and spontaneous pregnancy after combined heterotopic and orthotopic cryopreserved ovarian tissue transplantation in a patient previously treated with bone marrow transplantation: case report. Hum Reprod 21(8):2010–2014
36. Kim SS, Hwang IT, Lee HC (2004) Heterotopic autotransplantation of cryobanked human ovarian tissue as a strategy to restore ovarian function. Fertil Steril 82(4):930–932
37. Kim SS, Lee WS, Chung MK, Lee HC, Lee HH, Hill D (2009) Long-term ovarian function and fertility after heterotopic autotransplantation of cryobanked human ovarian tissue: 8-year experience in cancer patients. Fertil Steril 91(6):2349–2354
38. Kim SS (2012) Assessment of long term endocrine function after transplantation of frozen-thawed human ovarian tissue to the heterotopic site: 10 year longitudinal follow-up study. J Assist Reprod Genet 29(6):489–493
39. Stern CJ, Gook D, Hale LG, Agresta F, Oldham J, Rozen G et al (2013) First reported clinical pregnancy following heterotopic grafting of cryopreserved ovarian tissue in a woman after a bilateral oophorectomy. Hum Reprod 28(11):2996–2999
40. Stern CJ, Toledo MG, Hale LG, Gook DA, Edgar DH (2011) The first Australian experience of heterotopic grafting of cryopreserved ovarian tissue: evidence of establishment of normal ovarian function. Aust N Z J Obstet Gynaecol 51(3):268–275
41. Oktay K, Buyuk E, Veeck L, Zaninovic N, Xu K, Takeuchi T, Opsahl M, Rosenwaks Z (2004) Embryo development after heterotopic transplantation of cryopreserved ovarian tissue. Lancet. 363(9412):837–40
42. Oktay K (2006) Spontaneous conceptions and live birth after heterotopic ovarian transplantation:is there a germline stem cell connection? Hum Reprod 21(6):1345–8

43. Oktay K, Türkçüoğlu I, Rodriguez-Wallberg KA (2011) Four spontaneous pregnancies and three live births following subcutaneous transplantation of frozen banked ovarian tissue: what is the explanation? Fertil Steril. 95(2):804.e7-10
44. Schmidt KT, Rosendahl M, Ernst E, Loft A, Andersen AN, Dueholm M et al (2011) Autotransplantation of cryopreserved ovarian tissue in 12 women with chemotherapy-induced premature ovarian failure: the Danish experience. Fertil Steril 95(2):695–701
45. Demeestere I, Simon P, Emiliani S, Delbaere A, Englert Y (2007) Fertility preservation: successful transplantation of cryopreserved ovarian tissue in a young patient previously treated for Hodgkin's disease. Oncologist 12(12):1437–1442
46. Stern CJ, Gook D, Hale LG, Agresta F, Oldham J, Rozen G et al (2014) Delivery of twins following heterotopic grafting of frozen-thawed ovarian tissue. Hum Reprod 29(8):1828
47. Meirow D, Dor J, Kaufman B, Shrim A, Rabinovici J, Schiff E et al (2007) Cortical fibrosis and blood-vessels damage in human ovaries exposed to chemotherapy. Potential mechanisms of ovarian injury. Hum Reprod 22(6):1626–1633
48. Baird DT, Webb R, Campbell BK, Harkness LM, Gosden RG (1999) Long-term ovarian function in sheep after ovariectomy and transplantation of autografts stored at -196 C. Endocrinology 140(1):462–471
49. Liu J, Van der Elst J, Van den Broecke R, Dhont M (2002) Early massive follicle loss and apoptosis in heterotopically grafted newborn mouse ovaries. Hum Reprod 17(3):605–611
50. Newton H, Aubard Y, Rutherford A, Sharma V, Gosden R (1996) Low temperature storage and grafting of human ovarian tissue. Hum Reprod 11(7):1487–1491
51. Nisolle M, Casanas-Roux F, Qu J, Motta P, Donnez J (2000) Histologic and ultrastructural evaluation of fresh and frozen-thawed human ovarian xenografts in nude mice. Fertil Steril 74 (1):122–129
52. Nugent D, Newton H, Gallivan L, Gosden RG (1998) Protective effect of vitamin E on ischaemia-reperfusion injury in ovarian grafts. J Reprod Fertil 114(2):341–346
53. Israely T, Dafni H, Nevo N, Tsafriri A, Neeman M (2004) Angiogenesis in ectopic ovarian xenotransplantation: multiparameter characterization of the neovasculature by dynamic contrast-enhanced MRI. Magn Reson Med 52(4):741–750
54. Martinez-Madrid B, Donnez J, Van Eyck AS, Veiga-Lopez A, Dolmans MM, Van Langendonckt A (2009) Chick embryo chorioallantoic membrane (CAM) model: a useful tool to study short-term transplantation of cryopreserved human ovarian tissue. Fertil Steril 91 (1):285–292
55. Van Eyck AS, Jordan BF, Gallez B, Heilier JF, Van Langendonckt A, Donnez J (2009) Electron paramagnetic resonance as a tool to evaluate human ovarian tissue reoxygenation after xenografting. Fertil Steril 92(1):374–381
56. Van Eyck AS, Bouzin C, Feron O, Romeu L, Van Langendonckt A, Donnez J et al (2010) Both host and graft vessels contribute to revascularization of xenografted human ovarian tissue in a murine model. Fertil Steril 93(5):1676–1685
57. Soleimani R, Heytens E, Oktay K (2011) Enhancement of neoangiogenesis and follicle survival by sphingosine-1-phosphate in human ovarian tissue xenotransplants. PLoS One 6 (4):e19475
58. Suzuki H, Ishijima T, Maruyama S, Yanagimoto Ueta Y, Abe Y, Saitoh H (2008) Beneficial effect of desialylated erythropoietin administration on the frozen-thawed canine ovarian xenotransplantation. J Assist Reprod Genet 25(11–12):571–575
59. Commin L, Buff S, Rosset E, Galet C, Allard A, Bruyere P et al (2012) Follicle development in cryopreserved bitch ovarian tissue grafted to immunodeficient mouse. Reprod Fertil Dev 24 (3):461–471
60. Henry L, Labied S, Fransolet M, Kirschvink N, Blacher S, Noel A et al (2015) Isoform 165 of vascular endothelial growth factor in collagen matrix improves ovine cryopreserved ovarian tissue revascularisation after xenotransplantation in mice. Reprod Biol Endocrinol 13(1):12

61. Wang L, Ying YF, Ouyang YL, Wang JF, Xu J (2013) VEGF and bFGF increase survival of xenografted human ovarian tissue in an experimental rabbit model. J Assist Reprod Genet 30 (10):1301–1311
62. Callejo J, Salvador C, Gonzalez-Nunez S, Almeida L, Rodriguez L, Marques L et al (2013) Live birth in a woman without ovaries after autograft of frozen-thawed ovarian tissue combined with growth factors. J Ovarian Res 6(1):33
63. Wang H, Mooney S, Wen Y, Behr B, Polan ML (2002) Follicle development in grafted mouse ovaries after cryopreservation and subcutaneous transplantation. Am J Obstet Gynecol 187 (2):370–374
64. Weissman A, Gotlieb L, Colgan T, Jurisicova A, Greenblatt EM, Casper RF (1999) Preliminary experience with subcutaneous human ovarian cortex transplantation in the NOD-SCID mouse. Biol Reprod 60(6):1462–1467
65. Abir R, Fisch B, Jessel S, Felz C, Ben-Haroush A, Orvieto R (2011) Improving posttransplantation survival of human ovarian tissue by treating the host and graft. Fertil Steril 95(4):1205–1210
66. Sapmaz E, Ayar A, Celik H, Sapmaz T, Kilic N, Yasar MA (2003) Effects of melatonin and oxytetracycline in autologous intraperitoneal ovary transplantation in rats. Neuro Endocrinol Lett 24(5):350–354
67. Kim SS, Yang HW, Kang HG, Lee HH, Lee HC, Ko DS et al (2004) Quantitative assessment of ischemic tissue damage in ovarian cortical tissue with or without antioxidant (ascorbic acid) treatment. Fertil Steril 82(3):679–685
68. Fabbri R, Sapone A, Paolini M, Vivarelli F, Franchi P, Lucarini M et al (2015) Effects of N-acetylcysteine on human ovarian tissue preservation undergoing cryopreservation procedure. Histol Histopathol 30(6):725–735

Chapter 8
Sperm Cryopreservation

Takeshi Shin, Mai Fukushima, Akane Miyata, and Hiroshi Okada

Abstract Sperm cryopreservation, the preservation and storage of sperm for future use, is an efficient procedure for the management of male fertility and is now routinely offered to men as a means of preserving their fertility. Cryopreservation should be discussed and offered prior to cytotoxic therapy for not only malignant diseases but also nonmalignant systemic diseases such as autoimmune disorders or inflammatory bowel disease. There are many important steps in the process of successful cryopreservation. Freezing and thawing should be performed using techniques that minimize sperm damage. Although sperm banking is now a common technique all over the world, little has been written about the clinical process. In this chapter, we provide an overview of sperm cryopreservation, including its history and the methods used for cryopreservation. We also provide the indications of sperm cryopreservation and scientific background of the procedures.

Keywords Cryopreservation • Fertility preservation • History • Sperm

8.1 Introduction

Sperm cryopreservation is a method to preserve and store sperm for future use in assisted conception. Spermatozoa lose their cytoplasm during spermatogenesis. Because of the resulting decrease in water content, spermatozoa are more suitable for cryopreservation than eggs, embryos, or somatic cells. Currently, human sperm cryopreservation is widely used to preserve male fertility for assisted reproductive treatments, for example, by collecting sperm before chemotherapy, radiotherapy, or any surgery that would affect male reproductive systems. Because cancer cure rates have dramatically improved recently, "oncofertility," which is a new field of medicine, has emerged to focus on fertility preservation for cancer survivors. In addition, the recent development of assisted reproductive technology (ART) has expanded the needs for sperm cryopreservation. The need for sperm cryopreservation is expected

T. Shin (✉) • M. Fukushima • A. Miyata • H. Okada
Center for Reproductive Medicine, Dokkyo Medical University Koshigaya Hospital, 2-1-50 Minamikoshigaya, Koshigaya, Saitama 343-8555, Japan
e-mail: shintakeshi@nifty.com

N. Suzuki, J. Donnez (eds.), *Gonadal Tissue Cryopreservation in Fertility Preservation*, DOI 10.1007/978-4-431-55963-4_8

to continue, so we must seek to develop high-quality cryopreservation methods. In this chapter, we provide an overview of the history of sperm cryopreservation as well as its indications and methods.

8.2 History of Sperm Cryopreservation

Cryopreservation of sperm dates back to 1776 (Table 8.1). At that time Lazzaro Spallanzani first reported that sperm cooled by snow became motionless [1]. In 1866, Mantegazza, an Italian physician, observed survival of human spermatozoa that had been cooled to −150 °C and proposed the concept of a human sperm bank to store semen specimens [2]. However, it was not until the development of artificial insemination (AI) in the late 1950s that sperm cryopreservation became a major area of scientific investigation [3].

In the late 1930s and early 1940s, many researchers found that sperm could survive freezing to temperatures below −160 °C, but survival was limited in the absence of a cryoprotectant [1]. In 1949, Polge et al. made a significant discovery that the use of glycerol could protect sperm at low temperatures [4]. This was the defining moment in the establishment of sperm cryobiology. The discovery of glycerol as a cryoprotectant soon led to successful cryopreservation of bull sperm [5].

The first human pregnancies with frozen sperm were reported in 1953, when Bunge and Sherman froze human sperm with 10 % glycerol on dry ice and reported three pregnancies following AI with the thawed sperm [6]. The announcement, made at the 11th International Congress of Genetics in 1963, triggered interest in the possibility of sperm banks. After this report, many scientists began working toward sperm cryopreservation as a treatment for infertility. In the early 1960s, a method for freezing human semen in liquid nitrogen (LN_2) vapor and storing it at −196 °C was introduced. Sherman had discovered that storage of human sperm at −196 °C was superior to storage at −75 °C [7]. Storing human sperm in LN_2 has since become the standard. Clinical applications of cryobanking developed with the wider use of AI with husband, partner, or donor semen in the early 1970s [1].

Table 8.1 The history of sperm cryopreservation

Year	Event
1776	First observation of human sperm cooled by snow [1, 7]
1866	First proposal of the concept of a human sperm bank [1, 7]
1938	−269 °C survival; storage at −79 °C [7]
1949	Discovery of glycerol as a cryoprotective agent [4]
1951	First successful preservation of bull sperm [5]
1953	First successful human pregnancy using frozen-thawed sperm [6]
1962–1963	Sperm frozen and stored using liquid nitrogen [7]
1970s	Commercial sperm banks founded

The recent development of ART such as intracytoplasmic sperm injection (ICSI) has expanded the indications for sperm banking, and human sperm cryopreservation has become a routine procedure in ART laboratories.

8.3 Indications for Sperm Cryopreservation

Cryopreservation of sperm is mandatory in donor insemination programs. Donor sperm are used for couples in which the male partner has incurable male infertility or couples that wish to prevent transmission of a genetic or infectious disease from the male partner to the offspring. Donor sperm are also used for single women planning to become mothers and in several other circumstances in which fertility could be compromised. When AI is performed, insemination with the husband's or partner's sperm is generally performed with a fresh specimen; however, cryopreserved semen can be used in the case of irregular female cycles.

As described below, except for donor insemination, indications for sperm cryopreservation are mainly divided into two categories: fertility preservation and male infertility treatment (Table 8.2).

8.3.1 Sperm Cryopreservation as Fertility Preservation

8.3.1.1 Prior to Treatment for Malignancies

Cryopreservation should be discussed and offered prior to therapy for malignant diseases. The most common cancers that affect males of reproductive age include

Table 8.2 Indications for sperm banking (Modified from Hamada et al. [8])

	Patient condition	Sperm collection method
Fertility preservation	Cancer	Ejaculation
		Testicular tissue freezing in prepubertal boys
	Nonmalignant systemic disease	Ejaculation
	Prior to surgical procedure to treat or induce infertility	Ejaculation
	Occupational risk	Ejaculation
	Sex change	Ejaculation
		Testicular tissue freezing in male-to-female surgery
Fertility treatment	Azoospermia	Surgical retrieval techniques from testes or epididymis
	Severe oligozoospermia	Ejaculation
	Anejaculation	Assisted ejaculation
		Surgical retrieval techniques from testes or epididymis

Table 8.3 Indications for sperm banking in cancer patients

Cause of fertility loss	Disease or treatment
Loss of seminiferous tubules	Orchiectomy for bilateral testicular cancer
Spermatogenic dysfunction	Chemotherapy
	Radiotherapy
Loss of sperm delivery system	Urinary diversion for bladder cancer
Ejaculatory dysfunction	Surgery for colon cancer, bladder cancer, soft tissue tumor in pelvis
	Retroperitoneal lymph node dissection for testicular cancer

testicular cancer, acute leukemia, Hodgkin's disease, non-Hodgkin's lymphoma, and soft tissue tumors [9]. The recent advances in cancer therapies for males of pediatric, adolescent, and reproductive ages over the last several decades have led to increases in long-term survival, making posttreatment quality of life increasingly important [3]. Combinations of surgery, radiation therapy, and chemotherapy may achieve high remission rates in patients with cancer, but the treatment can be harmful to male fertility. Cytotoxic chemotherapy, radiotherapy, and some kinds of surgical treatment may lead to irreversible spermatogenic dysfunction, ejaculatory dysfunction, or unreconstructable obstruction [1] (Table 8.3). Cryopreservation of sperm before the initiation of treatment provides patients with future fertility potential. Cancer patients of reproductive age are most commonly referred to sperm banks in the United States [10].

Chemotherapeutic agents and irradiation specifically affect spermatogenesis. Among the germ cells, the differentiating spermatogonia proliferate most rapidly and undergo apoptosis. Because of this rapid division, differentiating spermatogonia are more sensitive to killing by radiation and cytotoxic chemotherapeutic drugs than the later-stage germ cells [11, 12], which are relatively resistant to killing but are sensitive to genetic damage. The spermatogonial stem cells appear to be more resistant to killing by cytotoxic therapies than the differentiating spermatogonia and are more sensitive than the later-stage germ cells. Thus, the surviving later-stage germ cells progress along their differentiation but are not replaced by new cells that would have been derived from the differentiating spermatogonia that had been killed [12].

During the first 2 months of cytotoxic chemotherapy, sperm counts may be only moderately reduced [13, 14]. Azoospermia appears 2 or 3 months after the initiation of therapy, which is the time required for differentiating spermatogonia to become sperm [14]. This induced azoospermia may be either transient or permanent. The recovery of spermatogenesis depends on the survival of the spermatogonial stem cells, and it depends on the nature and dose of the cytotoxic agent. Cisplatin and alkylating agents, such as nitrogen mustard, cyclophosphamide, ifosfamide, busulfan, procarbazine, and chlorambucil, are toxic to stem cells and can produce persistent azoospermia [14] (Table 8.4). These agents may also induce genetic damage by cross-linking DNA and introducing single-strand DNA breaks.

Table 8.4 Chemotherapeutic agents that can cause azoospermia (Slightly modified from Meistrich [14])

Effect	Agent	Cumulative dose for effect
Cause persistent azoospermia	Chlorambucil	1.4 g/m^2
	Cyclophosphamide	19 g/m^2
	Procarbazine	4 g/m^2
	Melphalan	140 mg/m^2
	Cisplatin	500 mg/m^2
Cause persistent azoospermia but always given with other highly sterilizing agents	Busulfan	600 mg/m^2
	Ifosfamide	42 g/m^2
	Nitrogen mustard	–
	Actinomycin D	–
Cause temporary reductions in sperm count when not combined with the above agents	Adriamycin	770 mg/m^2
	Thiotepa	400 mg/m^2
	Cytosine arabinoside	1 g/m^2
	Vinblastine	50 mg/m^2

Radiotherapy is similarly detrimental to spermatogenesis. The degree by which spermatogenesis is affected depends on the dosage. Doses above 0.15 Gy appear to reduce sperm count. Doses between 0.15 Gy and 0.5 Gy cause oligozoospermia [14]. The nadir of sperm count occurs 4–6 months after the treatment, and 10–18 months are required for complete recovery [15]. At doses of 0.6 Gy, reversible azoospermia occurs [14]. Radiation-induced temporary alterations in spermatogenesis may disappear within 2 years. Doses of 4 Gy appear to be the threshold for permanent azoospermia [16]. The detrimental effects are increased when chemotherapy and radiotherapy are used in combination [17]. Radiotherapy also causes sperm DNA fragmentation.

8.3.1.2 Prior to Treatment for Nonmalignant Diseases

Cryopreservation of sperm is recommended for men with nonmalignant systemic disease or treatment regimens which may cause infertility [18]. For example, men with autoimmune disorders, inflammatory bowel disease, kidney disorders, or hematologic diseases that are treated with bone marrow transplants may consider sperm banking early in the disease process because most of these patients require immunosuppressive or cytotoxic therapy. Men with these conditions should be made aware of the possible adverse effects of their disease on spermatogenesis and future ability to father a child. Although the pretreatment quality of semen in these men is inferior to that of healthy donors [18], sufficient viable sperm are present in the frozen-thawed specimen for ART [1].

8.3.1.3 Prior to Surgical Infertility Treatment

Sperm can be frozen before certain surgeries that are performed to cure infertility, such as varicocele ligation in men with severe oligozoospermia and surgical relief of seminal duct obstruction. These surgeries may be complicated postoperatively by testicular artery injury or inadvertent vas deferens transection. In these cases, preoperative sperm banking provides insurance in case azoospermia ensues post-operatively [1]. Fertility preservation may also be an option for men planning bilateral vasectomy for contraception, as they may change their mind regarding having children in the future.

8.3.1.4 Other Situations

Sperm banking is indicated for biological males who are planning sex reassignment through hormonal or surgical therapy. Estrogen has detrimental effects on spermatogenesis [19], and male-to-female sex change surgery including orchiectomy and penectomy renders the male sterile. After surgery, two-thirds of patients identify as lesbian [8], and some patients want to have children with their partners. Sperm cryopreservation before the sex change offers a chance for these couples to have children [8].

Cryopreservation of sperm is also recommended for men who work with toxic chemicals, ionization radiation, or biological hazards, because these exposures may have adverse effects on the reproductive system [8, 20].

Finally, men working in defense or security may have to face life-threatening situations and can avail themselves of cryopreservation before going to the battlefield.

8.3.2 Sperm Cryopreservation as Infertility Treatment

This group includes men with azoospermia, severe oligozoospermia, and ejaculatory dysfunction.

8.3.2.1 Azoospermia

Azoospermia is defined by the complete absence of spermatozoa in centrifuged semen samples collected on at least two occasions [21]. Azoospermia is typically classified into obstructive azoospermia and azoospermia due to spermatogenic dysfunction (ASD), formerly known as nonobstructive azoospermia. Because obstructive azoospermia is characterized by normal spermatogenesis but impaired sperm transport from the testes to the urethra, viable sperm can be obtained through various methods from the testes or epididymides. In contrast, ASD involves intratesticular defects in sperm production. Testicular sperm extraction (TESE) or microsurgical TESE are the preferred methods for obtaining sperm for men with ASD [22]. Cryopreservation of sperm obtained from testes or epididymides may obviate the need for repeated invasive sperm-harvesting procedures [1]. Preservation of sperm also allows ovarian stimulation of the female partner to be timed and eliminates the possibility of not finding sperm on the day of egg retrieval [1, 23, 24].

8.3.2.2 Severe Oligozoospermia

Severe oligozoospermia is defined by a very low sperm count of less than five million per milliliter [8]. Cryopreservation of existing spermatozoa ensures an adequate sperm supply for multiple ART cycles and avoids the expense and frustration of having an ICSI cycle end unsatisfactorily with no sperm in the ejaculate on the day of egg retrieval. Furthermore, recent reports have shown that some patients with severe oligozoospermia will become azoospermic [8, 25]. Male patients diagnosed with severe oligozoospermia should be informed about possible reduction of their residual spermatogenesis function and the necessity of intermittent follow-up semen analyses. If follow-up semen tests show declines in spermatogenesis, sperm cryopreservation may be recommended for these patients [26].

8.3.2.3 Ejaculatory Dysfunction

Sperm banking is recommended for men with anejaculation. Most men with spinal cord injury have ejaculatory dysfunction. For these patients, sperm ejaculated by penile vibrator or electroejaculation, or surgically obtained sperm from the testes or epididymides, should be cryopreserved for multiple ART cycles.

8.4 Process of Cryopreservation

There are many important stages for successful cryopreservation (Fig. 8.1), and technical or managerial errors at any stage can adversely affect the final outcome. In particular, freezing and thawing should be performed using methods that minimize sperm damage. This section highlights the key points at each step of the process.

8.4.1 Screening for Infectious Disease

All sperm donors are required to complete a screening with blood tests for human immunodeficiency virus (HIV), human T-lymphotropic virus (HTLV), hepatitis B

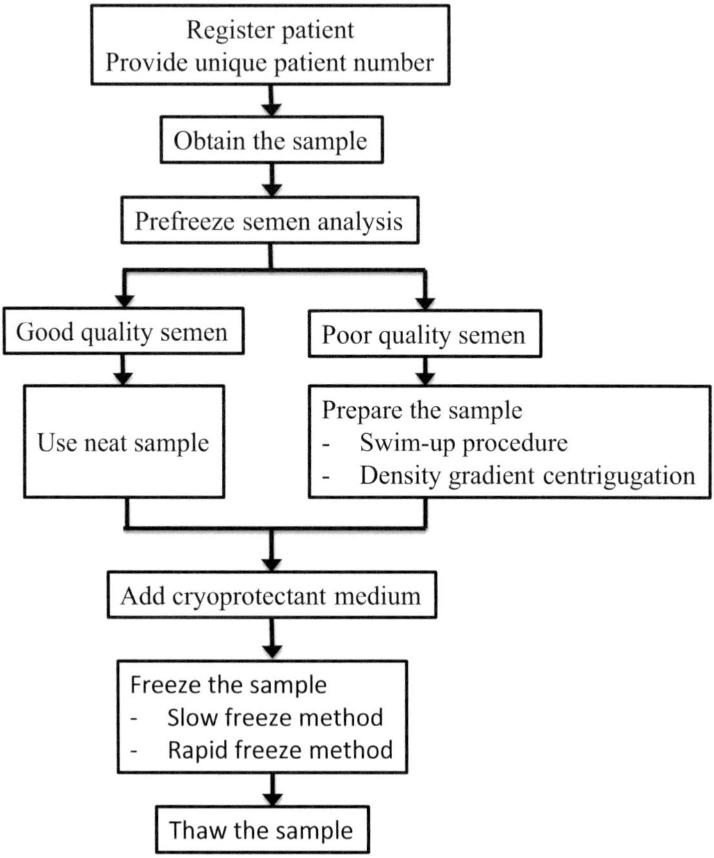

Fig. 8.1 Flowchart illustrating the stages of sperm banking

virus (HBV), hepatitis C virus (HCV), syphilis, and sometimes cytomegalovirus [8]. HIV, HCV, HBV, and possibly other viruses can survive in LN_2, making it possible to cross-contaminate samples in LN_2 storage tanks. Although there is no documentation of cross-contamination of stored human tissue, the American Society for Reproductive Medicine recommends that semen from patients infected with HIV, HCV, and/or HBV should be stored in separate storage tanks because of the theoretic risk of transmission [27].

8.4.2 Semen Analysis

Semen is first analyzed for parameters such as adequate sperm count, motility, and morphology. A computerized assisted semen analyzer can be used to provide additional information about the kinetic properties of semen before freezing and after thawing [8]. For diagnostic purposes, acceptance criteria for ejaculate specimens are that analysis begins within an hour of its production after at least 2 days of sexual abstinence [21]. However, patients facing lifesaving cytotoxic therapy do not necessarily adhere to such standards [28].

8.4.3 Sperm-Washing Procedure

Many sperm banks store masturbatory ejaculates in their raw state. The benefit of using unprocessed semen is that the natural antioxidant enzymes and scavenging molecules are still present to protect against free radical damage during freezing [8, 29]. However, given the high incidence of poor semen quality among cancer patients and infertile men, some prefer to subject semen samples to washing procedures before the samples are frozen [8]. Sperm washing is the primary procedure for separating sperm from seminal plasma, with the goals of removing decapacitation factors and other detrimental elements and concentrating all sperm within the ejaculate. Some authors have demonstrated clearly superior post-thaw outcomes after the use of sperm-washing methods [30, 31]. Moreover, the removal of any contaminating pathogens, such as HIV, from the seminal fluid by sperm washing is a secure way to reduce the likelihood of a cross-infection incident within a freezer [28]. For these reasons, sperm washing before cryopreservation is strongly recommended. Nonetheless, most sperm banks perform cryopreservation of neat semen.

There are two broad ways to classify sperm-washing protocols: the swim-up technique and the density-gradient method. In the swim-up procedure, a layer of an appropriate culture medium is gently added to the semen sample in such a way that most of the motile sperm will swim out of the sample and upward into the added medium. These harvested motile sperm are aspirated, centrifuged, and resuspended again to be stored. This procedure takes 2 hours. In the density-gradient method, different concentrations of solutions (colloidal silica and a tri-iodinated derivative of benzoic acid) are layered in a test tube in ascending order of density (heaviest layer at the bottom). When a semen sample is placed upon the uppermost isolate layer and centrifuged for 30 minutes, any debris, round cells, and nonmotile and poor-quality sperm remain in the top layers. Only the highly motile sperm are able to get through to the bottom layer. Sperm pellets are resuspended in an appropriate medium and prepared for the next step.

8.4.4 Techniques for Cryopreservation

Compared to embryo or egg freezing, the cryopreservation of sperm is relatively crude. To date, there are three main freezing techniques used in cryopreservation: slow freezing, rapid freezing, and vitrification. Most sperm banks still freeze sperm by the method of rapid freezing first reported by Sherman, which involves suspending semen samples in nitrogen vapor for a period of time before plunging them into LN_2 [28]. Figure 8.2 shows our cryopreservation protocol.

8.4.4.1 Slow Freezing

Behrman and Sawada introduced the slow-freezing technique that cools sperm progressively over a period of 2–4 hours [32]. It allows the sperm cells to gradually adjust to cold conditions, and it places less osmotic strain on the cellular membrane than rapid freezing does [8]. Cooling is performed either manually or automatically using a programmable freezer. The manual method is performed by simultaneously decreasing the temperature of the sample while adding a cryoprotectant in a stepwise manner [33]. The optimal initial cooling rate of the sample from room temperature to 5 °C is 0.5–1 °C/min [33, 34]. The sample is then frozen from 5 °C to −80 °C at a rate of 1–10 °C/min before it is plunged into LN_2 [33]. Computer-controlled freezers provide advantages above the manual methods with regard to validation and consistency [28]. In most programmable freezers, the straws or vials are cooled by cold nitrogen vapor. The temperature inside the cooling chamber can be accurately controlled, and the time course of the temperature can be programmed. Careful monitoring of the rate of freezing helps to prevent rapid cellular dehydration and ice crystal formation. However, conventional slow freezing, either manual or automated, may cause extensive chemical and physical damage to the sperm because of ice crystallization [35].

8.4.4.2 Rapid Freezing

Rapid freezing minimizes the toxicity of the cryoprotectant and reduces osmotic membrane damage due to the formation of extracellular ice crystals [8]. This method was first introduced by Sherman [28]. Here we describe a variation on Sherman's method. The samples are initially mixed in a dropwise manner with an equal volume of cryoprotectant. They are placed in vials or straws and then in nitrogen vapor at −96 °C for 2 hours. There is a thermal gradient within the vapor that depends on the volume of the liquid nitrogen in the tank and the distance of the sample from it [33]. The samples are finally immersed in LN_2 at −196 °C. Rapid freezing leads to better post-thaw motility and survival than slow freezing [36]. However, Fabbri et al. pointed out that the cooling temperature curve cannot be controlled, and the freezing temperature might vary [33].

8.4.4.3 Vitrification

In 1984, the combination of rapid cooling and high cryoprotectant concentration to completely avoid ice formation was first suggested by Fahy et al. [37]. This

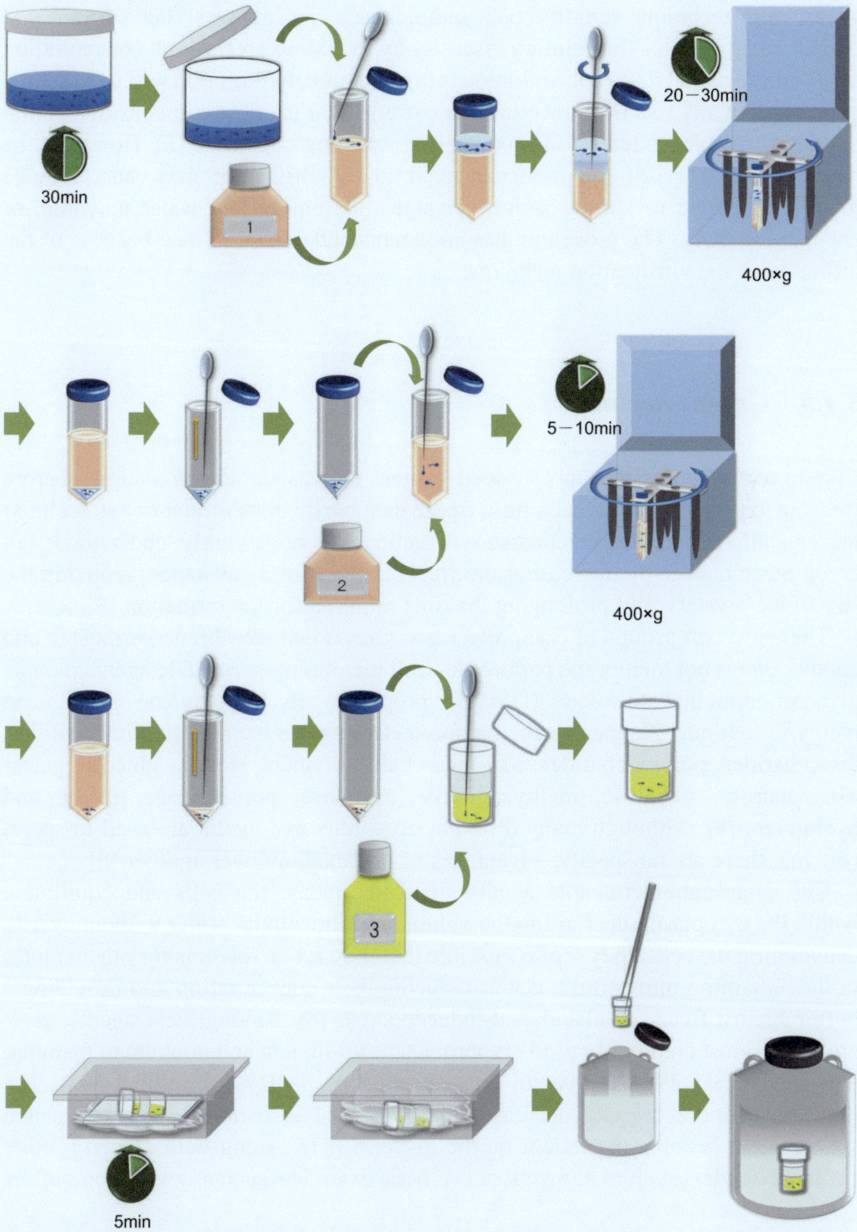

Fig. 8.2 Sperm-freezing protocol in our laboratory (medium 1, density-gradient centrifugation medium; medium 2, sperm-washing medium; medium 3, cryoprotective medium). (1) Allow specimen to liquefy at room temperature completely for 30 minutes before processing. (2) Layer the liquefied semen onto the density-gradient centrifugation medium. (3) Centrifuge at 400 × g for 20–30 min. (4) Aspirate in a circular movement from the surface everything except the pellet. If no pellet is seen after centrifugation, remove all fluid except the lowest 0.5 mL. (5) Use a new pipette to aspirate the pellet (or the lowest 0.5 mL). Transfer sperm pellet to a new tube and re-suspend pellet in sperm-washing medium. (6) Centrifuge at 400 × g for 5–10 minutes. (7) Aspirate sperm-

vitrification technique rapidly cools samples at a rate of over 1000 °C/min and dramatically elevates the solution viscosity by including a very high concentration of cryoprotectants; if the concentration is high enough, the solution will solidify to a glass without any risk of intracellular or extracellular ice formation during cooling or warming, independent of the cooling and warming rates used [8]. However, the high concentrations of cryoprotectant required for vitrification may cause damage to the sperm due to abrupt osmotic changes, extremely low water potential, or chemical toxicity. The procedure has not been standardized to date because of the difficulty of the vitrification technique.

8.4.5 Cryoprotectants

Cryoprotectants are substances added to neat or washed semen samples before freezing to protect spermatozoa from freeze damage by intracellular or extracellular ice crystallization. The mechanisms of action are not entirely understood, but cryoprotectants act by decreasing the freezing point of a substance, reducing the size of ice crystals, and prolonging the time required for ice formation [8].

There are two groups of cryoprotectants. One is cell membrane permeable and another one is not membrane permeable. Cell membrane-permeable agents include glycerol, dimethyl sulfoxide (DMSO), propylene glycol, ethylene glycol, and methylformamide. Nonpermeable cryoprotective agents include monosaccharides, disaccharides, polysaccharides, and long-chain polymers, such as glucose, galactose, sucrose, trehalose, methylcellulose, raffinose, polyethylene glycol, and hyaluronan [8]. Although many different cryoprotective media are used in sperm banking, there are no specific advantages of one medium over another [8].

Cell membrane-permeable agents slowly permeate the cells and equilibrate within the cytoplasm, decreasing the volume of intracellular water without overtly dehydrating the cell. They are so miscible that they act as solvents for other solutes in the remaining intracellular water, reducing their concentration and providing a buffer against freezing-related, salt-induced stress [8]. Among these agents, glycerol is the most commonly used cryoprotectant for human and nonhuman mammalian sperm [38, 39]. A glycerol concentration of 5–10 % is optimal [40]. The motility of sperm rapidly decreases after glycerol is removed, suggesting that sperm might become dependent on the glycerol [41]. Along with glycerol, other natural extenders such as egg yolk or synthetic extenders such as zwitterion buffers

---

Fig. 8.2 (continued) washing medium supernatant leaving as little liquid as possible above the pellet. If no pellet is seen, leave the bottom 0.25 mL fluid. (8) Transfer specimen from a centrifuge pipette to a cryovial. (9) Cryoprotective medium is added until a defined ratio of semen sample to medium is achieved. (10) The cryovials were capped and placed into liquid nitrogen vapor for cooling 5 minutes. (11) Frozen samples in the cryovial are transferred and stored in liquid nitrogen storage tank

containing tris (hydroxymethyl) aminomethane, N-tris (hydroxymethyl) methyl-2-aminoethanesulfonic acid (TES), or a combination of these are generally used routinely for better recovery of motile sperm [42, 43].

Although nonpermeable agents are unable to permeate the plasma membrane, these agents can stabilize the lipid bilayer, forming hydrogen bonds between hydrophilic sides. They increase viscosity and lower the freezing point of the extracellular fluid even though they promote fast cellular dehydration [8]. Egg yolk, milk, soy lecithin, and albumin are also considered nonpermeable cryoprotective agents; they protect sperm membranes from cold injury, although the mechanism of protection is unknown. These high-molecular-weight cryoprotectants are included in every cryoprotective medium and used synergistically with permeable cryoprotectants to reduce the toxic concentration of the permeable cryoprotectants [8].

8.4.6 Containment System

The containment system used to store a patient's sperm is important. Semen samples are generally stored in cryovials or plastic straws. Cryovials have been extensively used for storing sperm, particularly since the mid-1990s [28]. They are made of plastic material with either polypropylene or polyethylene screw caps. Filling and labeling is easier with cryovials than with straws. However, uniform cooling of the sample is impossible to achieve because of the relatively large diameters and semen volumes. Furthermore, during cooling the vials shrink and are embrittled, and the contents create a vacuum that permits LN_2 to be drawn into the vials. The use of cryovials should be limited to vapor-phase storage only [28]. In contrast, straws or paillettes are small-radius tubes that provide a uniform cooling system. These were developed for the veterinary industry and originally made from polyvinyl chloride (PVC) and are now made from polyethylene terephthalate glycol (PETG) [44]. PVC straws were withdrawn in 1998, because the PVC disintegrated under radiation sterilization. PETG straws can hold 0.25–0.5 mL of semen and are usually sealed from both ends by ultrasonic welding, solid plastic plugs, or hematocrit tube sealant. Air space must be left to allow for expansion during cooling [8]. Table 8.5 summarizes the advantages and disadvantages of the packing systems.

Table 8.5 Relative advantages of the two packaging systems for freezing sperm

	Cryovials	PETG straws
Uniform cooling	+	+++
Available in small, convenient units	+++	+++
Robust at −196 °C	+++	+
Suitable for immersion in LN_2	+	++
Easy to label clearly	+++	+

8.4.7 Thawing Procedure

The thawing procedure is an equally important step. It must be performed carefully to minimize sperm damage, and abrupt thermal changes should be avoided as far as possible to enable sperm to recover their normal biological activities. Generally, the cryopreservation protocols use a thawing temperature of 37 °C [33]. In the first step, the cryovial or straw is placed at room temperature for several minutes and then in a water bath at 37 °C for 10–20 minutes. In the second step, the cryoprotective agent is slowly removed from the cells using sperm-washing medium.

References

1. Anger JT, Gilbert BR, Goldstein M (2003) Cryopreservation of sperm: indications, methods and results. J Urol 170:1079–1084
2. Bunge RG, Keettel WC, Sherman JK (1954) Clinical use of frozen semen: report of four cases. Fertil Steril 5:520–529
3. Walters EM, Benson JD, Woods EJ et al (2009) The history of sperm cryopreservation. In: Pacey AA, Tomlinson M (eds) Sperm banking theory and practice. Cambridge University Press, London, pp 1–17
4. Polge C, Smith AU, Parkes AS (1949) Revival of spermatozoa after vitrification and dehydration at low temperatures. Nature 164:666
5. Polge C (1952) Fertilizing capacity of bull spermatozoa after freezing at −79°C. Nature 169:626–627
6. Bunge RG, Sherman JK (1953) Fertilizing capacity of frozen human spermatozoa. Nature 172:767–768
7. Sherman JK (1980) Historical synopsis of human semen cryobanking. In: David G, Price WS (eds) Human artificial insemination and semen preservation. Springer, New York, pp 95–105
8. Hamada A, Wasik M, Gupta S et al (2012) Sperm banking: indications and regulations. In: Dubey AK (ed) Infertility: diagnosis, management and IVF. Jaypee Brothers Medical Publishing, New Delhi, pp 409–434
9. Sabanegh ES Jr, Ragheb AM (2009) Male fertility after cancer. Urology 73:225–231
10. Tomlinson M (2010) Therapeutic sperm cryopreservation. In: Björndahl L, Giwercman A, Tournaye L (eds) Clinical andrology EAU/ESAU course guidelines. Informa Health Care, London, pp 124–133
11. Meistrich ML, Finch M, da Cunha MF et al (1982) Damaging effects of fourteen chemotherapeutic drugs on mouse testis cells. Cancer Res 42:122–131
12. Sigman M (2013) Cancer treatment and male infertility: effects of therapy and current and future management options. Fertil Steril 100:1179–1186
13. Meistrich ML, Wilson G, Mathur K et al (1997) Rapid recovery of spermatogenesis after mitoxantrone, vincristine, vinblastine, and prednisone chemotherapy for Hodgkin's disease. J Clin Oncol 15:3488–3495
14. Meistrich ML (2009) Effect of antineoplastic and other medical treatments on sperm production. In: Pacey AA, Tomlinson M (eds) Sperm banking theory and practice. Cambridge University Press, London, pp 18–29
15. Gordon W, Siegmund K, Stanisic TH et al (1997) A study of reproductive function in patients with seminoma treated with radiotherapy and orchidectomy: (SWOG-8711). Int J Radiat Oncol Biol Phys 38:83–94

16. Wallace WH (2011) Oncofertility and preservation of reproductive capacity in children and young adults. Cancer 117:2301–2310
17. Colpi GM, Contalbi GF, Nerva F et al (2004) Testicular function following chemo-radiotherapy. Eur J Obstet Gynecol Reprod Biol 113:S2–S6
18. Ranganathan P, Mahran AM, Hallak J et al (2002) Sperm cryopreservation for men with nonmalignant, systemic diseases: a descriptive study. J Androl 23:71–75
19. Mishra DP, Shaha C (2005) Estrogen-induced spermatogenic cell apoptosis occurs via the mitochondrial pathway: role of superoxide and nitric oxide. J Biol Chem 280:6181–6196
20. Gupta S, Agarwal A, Sharma R (2011) Recovery, preparation, storage and utilization of spermatozoa for fertility preservation in cancer patients and subfertile men. J Reprod Stem Cell Biotechnol 1:150–168
21. World Health Organization, Department of Reproductive Health and Research (2010) WHO laboratory manual for the examination and processing of human semen, 5th edn.
22. Okada H, Dobashi M, Yamazaki T et al (2002) Conventional versus microdissection testicular sperm extraction for nonobstructive azoospermia. J Urol 168:1063–1067
23. Marmar JL (1998) The emergence of specialized procedures for the acquisition, processing, and cryopreservation of epididymal and testicular sperm in connection with intracytoplasmic sperm injection. J Androl 19:517–526
24. Kupker W, Schlegel PN, Al-Hasani S et al (2000) Use of frozen-thawed testicular sperm for intracytoplasmic sperm injection. Fertil Steril 73:453–458
25. Bak CW, Song SH, Yoon TK et al (2010) Natural course of idiopathic oligozoospermia: comparison of mild, moderate and severe forms. Int J Urol 17:937–943
26. Song SH, Bak CW, Lim JJ et al (2010) Natural course of severe oligozoospermia in infertile male: influence on future fertility potential. J Androl 31:536–539
27. Practice Committee of American Society for Reproductive Medicine (2013) Recommendations for reducing the risk of viral transmission during fertility treatment with the use of autologous gametes: a committee opinion. Fertil Steril 99:340–346
28. Tomlinson MJ (2009) Sperm processing and storage. In: Pacey AA, Tomlinson M (eds) Sperm banking theory and practice. Cambridge University Press, London, pp 86–104
29. Kalthur G, Adiga SK, Upadhya D et al (2008) Effect of cryopreservation on sperm DNA integrity in patients with teratospermia. Fertil Steril 89:1723–1727
30. Sherma RK, Agarwal A (1997) Influence of artificial stimulation on unprocessed and Percoll-washed cryopreserved sperm. Arch Androl 38:173–179
31. Esteves SC, Sharma RK, Thomas AJ Jr et al (2000) Improvement in motion characteristics and acrosome status in cryopreserved human spermatozoa by swim-up processing before freezing. Human Reprod 15:2173–2179
32. Behrman SJ, Sawada Y (1966) Heterologous and homologous inseminations with human semen frozen and stored in a liquid-nitrogen refrigerator. Fertil Steril 17:457–466
33. Di Santo M, Tarozzi N, Nadalini M et al (2012) Human sperm cryopreservation: update on techniques, effect on DNA integrity, and implications for ART. Adv Urol 2012:854837
34. Mahadevan M, Trounson AO (1984) Effect of cooling, freezing, and thawing rates and storage conditions on preservation of human spermatozoa. Andrologia 16:52–60
35. Mazur P, Rall WF, Rigopoulos N (1981) Relative contributions of the fraction of unfrozen water and of salt concentration to the survival of slowly frozen human erythrocytes. Biophys J 36:653–675
36. Nallella KP, Sharma RK, Allamaneni SS et al (2004) Cryopreservation of human spermatozoa: comparison of two cryopreservation methods and three cryoprotectants. Fertil Steril 82:913–918
37. Fahy GM, MacFarlane DR, Angell CA et al (1984) Vitrification as an approach to cryopreservation. Cryobiology 21:407–426
38. Cohen J, Garrisi GJ, Congedo-Ferrara TA et al (1997) Cryopreservation of single human spermatozoa. Hum Reprod 12:994–1001

39. Critser JK, Huse-Benda AR, Aaker DV et al (1988) Cryopreservation of human spermatozoa. III. The effect of cryoprotectants on motility. Fertil Steril 50:314–320
40. Hammitte DG, Walker DL, Williamson RA (1988) Concentration of glycerol required for optimal survival and in vitro fertilizing capacity of frozen sperm is dependent on cryopreservation medium. Fertil Steril 4:680–687
41. Jeyendran RS, Van der Ven MM, Kennedy W et al (1984) Comparison of glycerol and a zwitterion buffer system as cryoprotective media for human spermatozoa. J Androl 5:1–6
42. Jeyendran RS, Van der Ven MM, Kennedy W et al (1985) Effect of glycerol and cryopreservation on oocyte penetration by human spermatozoa. Andrologia 17:241–248
43. Puris GS, Weidel L (1986) A comparative study of buffer systems as cryoprotectants for human spermatozoa. Fertil Steril 46:147–149
44. Mortimer D (2004) Current and future concepts and practices in human sperm cryobanking. Reprod Biomed Online 9:134–151

Chapter 9
Testicular Tissue Cryopreservation

Herman Tournaye, Greta Verheyen, and Ellen Goossens

Abstract Loss of spermatogonial stem cells can be associated to ageing or can be part of genetic disorders such as 47,XXY Klinefelter syndrome. However, cytotoxic therapies and/or irradiation is the main cause of germ cell loss and can disrupt spermatogenesis temporarily or permanently. These therapies are not only used to treat malignant disorders but may also be used for benign haematological conditions that need bone-marrow transplantation.

Since survival rates after cancer treatment are increasing, preservation of the reproductive potential has become an important quality of life issue for both adults but also for childhood cancer survivors. Adult men who cannot bank ejaculate spermatozoa can opt to cryopreserve surgically retrieved spermatozoa, i.e. testicular sperm. Prepubertal boys cannot benefit from sperm banking, but testicular stem cell banking is being introduced into more and more clinics. This strategy should still be regarded as experimental given the lack of any report on successful transplantation and the limited safety data of this method.

Keywords Cancer • Spermatogonial stem cell • Cryopreservation • Klinefelter • Transplantation

---

H. Tournaye (✉)
Centre for Reproductive Medicine, Universitair Ziekenhuis Brussel, Vrije Universiteit Brussel, Laarbeeklaan 101, 1090 Brussels, Belgium

Research Group Biology of the Testis (BITE), Vrije Universiteit Brussel, Laarbeeklaan 103, 1090 Brussels, Belgium
e-mail: Tournaye@uzbrussel.be

G. Verheyen
Centre for Reproductive Medicine, Universitair Ziekenhuis Brussel, Vrije Universiteit Brussel, Laarbeeklaan 101, 1090 Brussels, Belgium

E. Goossens
Research Group Biology of the Testis (BITE), Vrije Universiteit Brussel, Laarbeeklaan 103, 1090 Brussels, Belgium

N. Suzuki, J. Donnez (eds.), *Gonadal Tissue Cryopreservation in Fertility Preservation*, DOI 10.1007/978-4-431-55963-4_9

9.1 Introduction

Spermatogenesis is the key to male fertility. From puberty onwards, spermatogonial stem cells will not only self-renew but also enter into a process of differentiation.

Spermatogonial stem cell self-renewal is promoted by several transcription factors, mainly regulated through the glial cell line-derived neurotropic factor (GDNF) [1, 2], but other transcription factors promoting self-renewal acting independently of GDNF control have also been described [2].

The pathways that promote differentiation are being investigated too, and it was shown that promyelocytic leukaemia zinc finger (Plzf) is a transcriptional repressor preventing differentiation of spermatogonial stem cells [3, 4]. Although the complex transcriptional network balancing self-renewal against differentiation is not fully understood, one may assume that spermatogonial stem cell loss can result from regulatory modifications in the molecular network. Specific genetic conditions such as 47,XXY Klinefelter syndrome are known to be associated to spermatogonial stem cell loss: at birth, Klinefelter patients have spermatogonial stem cells in their testes; however, during puberty self-renewal slows down and germ cells start to degenerate. The testes of adult Klinefelter patients are characterized by Sertoli cell-only tubules and massive fibrosis, although tubules with spermatogenesis can be found focally. Also, the presence of an Yq-deletion is assumed to be associated to gradual stem cell loss [5]. Gradual stem cell loss also occurs naturally with ageing. However, this natural spermatogonial stem cell loss is progressing very slowly, and only with older age (80–90 years old) all spermatogonial stem cells eventually disappear [6].

The most important cause for massive spermatogonial stem cell loss during the reproductive years is gonadotoxic treatment, i.e. chemotherapy and/or radiotherapy. Depending on the dose and the regimen applied, germ cells decrease in absolute numbers or completely disappear [7].

Given the better survival rates for many cancers, even cancers occurring in childhood, quality of life has become an important issue in cancer treatment [8]. While sperm banking is the golden standard to preserve male fertility in adult men undergoing potential sterilizing treatment [9], not all adult men present spermatozoa in their ejaculates when cancer is being diagnosed [10]. When cancer is diagnosed in childhood, active spermatogenesis is not present; hence cryobanking of spermatozoa is not an option.

When ejaculated spermatozoa cannot be cryopreserved, cryopreservation of testicular tissue either containing spermatozoa or spermatogonial stem cells may be considered.

9.2 Cryopreserving Testicular Tissue in Adults

If azoospermia is diagnosed in an adult man suffering from cancer, testicular spermatozoa can be obtained through a surgical procedure. In patients undergoing orchiectomy for testicular cancer, sperm can be aspirated from the vas deferens or from the epididymis [11], or from the testis [12, 13]. However, not only in men with testicular cancer spermatozoa can be obtained by testicular biopsy but also in men with other malignancies: testicular sperm has been extracted from biopsies of azoospermic men with malignant lymphomas [14]. This procedure was called onco-TESE (oncological testicular sperm extraction) and was reported to be successful in 8 out of 17 patients with malignant lymphoma [14, 15].

Testicular tissue cryopreservation containing spermatozoa is also an option for adolescents in whom ejaculated spermatozoa cannot be obtained [15]. Freezing of testicular cell suspensions preserves mature spermatozoa better than biopsy freezing.

The protocol currently used in our institution for cryopreserving testicular tissue containing spermatozoa can be found in the Appendix.

9.3 Testicular Tissue Cryopreservation in Boys

Before puberty, the only strategy to cope with spermatogonial stem cell loss and hence loss of the reproductive potential is the cryopreservation of testicular tissue containing spermatogonial stem cells.

In a mouse model, it has been shown that spermatogonial stem cells can be cryopreserved and install active spermatogenesis after infusion into the seminiferous tubules [16]. Today, numerous studies mainly performed in rodent models have been published, and therefore, cryopreservation of testicular tissue containing spermatogonial stem cells has been introduced in a few clinics worldwide [17].

From rodent models, we learn that two strategies can install spermatogenesis, i.e. transplantation of spermatogonial stem cells via infusion of the cell suspension into the seminiferous tubules [18] or grafting of frozen-thawed tissue [19].

Recently, successful spermatogonial stem cell transplantation has been reported in a primate model [20]. The results reported by Herman et al. indicated that active spermatogenesis could be obtained after transplanting spermatogonial stem cells in prepubertal but also adult rhesus monkeys that were chemotherapy treated before transplantation. Moreover, they showed that the spermatozoa obtained after transplantation were able to fertilize oocytes and generate cleaving embryos.

While testicular tissue freezing for spermatogonial stem cell transplantation is a very promising strategy in animal models, any clinical introduction in a human setting still needs further research. At present, no standardized cryopreservation protocol is available for banking testicular tissue in view of spermatogonial stem cell transplantation. The majority of centres preserving tissue use a controlled slow freezing protocol with the penetrating dimethyl sulfoxide (DMSO) combined with the non-permeating sucrose as the preferred cryoprotective agents [21]. This protocol is considered as being optimal based on histological and electron-microscopic studies as well as viability testing on the frozen-thawed tissue.

Recently, however, ultrarapid freezing protocols [22] and uncontrolled slow freezing protocols [23] have been introduced and were shown to be comparable to the slow freezing protocols which necessitate an expensive biofreezer. However, it remains essential to perform functionality assays with the frozen-thawed tissue. Only spermatogonial stem cell transplantation or tissue culture experiments can indicate which cryopreservation protocol has to be preferred as these are the only bioassays available to study both survival and functionality of spermatogonial stem cells.

The protocols currently used in our institution for cryopreserving prepubertal testicular tissue can be found in the Appendix.

Since the numbers of true spermatogonial stem cells in a small testicular tissue sample are limited, propagation of spermatogonial stem cells will be a crucial requisite for successful clinical introduction. In mice, it has been shown that spermatogonial stem cells can be cultured over 2 years and produce offspring after round spermatid injection and transfer to pseudopregnant recipient mice [24]. In the human too, in vitro culture and propagation of spermatogonial stem cells has been reported both with stem cells derived from adult testicular tissue and from tissue obtained from prepubertal boys [25, 26]. It was also shown that over a 50 days culture period, the spermatogonial stem cells did not show any increase of aneuploidy or epigenetic changes [27]. However, it should be noted that recent studies raise concerns about possible misinterpretation of these human SSC propagation data [28–31]. In mice, it was reported that offspring obtained after spermatogonial stem cell transplantation did not show any relevant epigenetic changes too [32–34].

Another important safety issue concerns cryopreservation and eventual transplantation of malignant cells, e.g. in boys with leukaemia. As it was demonstrated in a rat model that transmission of leukaemia by transplanting testicular cells is possible [35], elimination of malignant cells both by cell sorting [36] and by in vitro cultures [37] may lower or even circumvent the risk for reintroducing cancer via transplantation.

While many oncofertility programmes now start cryobanking testicular tissues also in prepubertal boys, there is still a debate on indications for banking. Given the fact that transplantational grafting of cryopreserved testicular tissue remains an experimental procedure, some programmes limit banking to boys with a high risk of sterility after chemotherapy. Although cryopreserving prepubertal testicular tissue is still being considered as an experimental procedure, a majority of parents of boys facing sterilizing cancer treatments already accepts this strategy in Western and non-Western societies [38–41].

Appendix

Protocol for Cryopreservation of Human Testicular Tissue (Containing Spermatozoa) in View of Fertility Preservation

Cryopreservation Medium ready for use sperm freezing medium based on glycerol, commercially available from different companies.

Collection Medium for Testicular Tissue Hepes-buffered HTF or sperm buffer supplemented with HSA, commercially available from different companies.

Preparation and Freezing of Testicular Tissue

1. Place the excised biopsies in a sterile petridish or tube filled with 5 ml of Hepes-buffered collection medium at room temperature and transport it to the laboratory
2. Unravel and mince the biopsies with the help of sterile pincettes, scissors or bended needles under the stereomicroscope in a laminar flow
3. Control the presence of spermatozoa in the suspension under the inverted microscope at 200× or 400× magnification
4. Put the suspension in a 10 ml Facon tube and centrifuge at 750 × g for 5 min
5. Discard the supernatant and resuspend the pellet in a volume which depends on the volume of the tissue
6. Add cryopreservation medium which was brought at room temperature dropwise, the volume to add depends on the volume of the final suspension and on the volume: volume ratio according to the manufacturer's instructions.
7. Aspirate the mixture in high-security straws, which are heat sealed.
8. Freezing is carried out in a programmable freezer with a programme for ejaculated sperm.
9. At the end of the programme, plunge the straws into LN2 and transport to and store in the LN2 container (vapour phase or liquid phase).

Protocol for Cryopreservation of Prepubertal Human Testicular Tissue (Spermatogonial Stem Cells) in View of Fertility Preservation

Components of the medium	Company and product N°	Storage
Hepes-buffered DMEM/F12	Gibco 31330-095	4 °C
HSA (human serum albumin)	Vitrolife 10064	4 °C
Sucrose	Sigma S1888-500G	RT
DMSO	WAK Chemie WAK-DMSO-10	RT

Fresh Preparation of the Cryopreservation Medium
2.55 g sucrose (0.15 M) + 40 ml DMEM/F12
→ in a sterile container, wait until sucrose dissolves, filter it
+5 ml HAS 10 %)
+5 ml sterile DMSO (1.5 M)
Keep on melting ice (4 °C) prior to use

Preliminary Preparation of the Cryopreservation Medium
2.55 g sucrose (0.15 M) + 40 ml DMEM/F12
→ in a sterile sperm container, wait until sucrose dissolves, filter it
→ aliquot 8 ml in Falcon tubes
→ store at −20 °C

Day of Use
Thaw one Falcon tube sucrose solution
+1 ml HSA (10 %) per Falcon tube
+1 ml sterile DMSO (1.5 M)
Keep on melting ice (4 °C) prior to use

Washing Medium
Hepes-buffered DMEM at 4 °C

Preparation and Freezing of Testicular Tissue

1. Clean the laminar flow, work as aseptic as possible.
2. The tissue is collected and transported in a sterile container with 0.9 % NaCl on ice. Take the tissue out of the collecting container.

   Transfer the tissue to a large sterile petridish containing DMEM. Work on ice water or use a cooling element.

   Rinse the tissue well.
3. Transfer the tissue to a second petridish containing DMEM on ice water/cooling element.
4. Cut the tissue in fragments of 6 mm^3 using a sterile scissor and pincet.

   Remove the tunica, if present.
5. Rinse the fragments in a third petridish containing DMEM on ice water/cooling element.
6. Reserve one of the fragments for histological analysis.

   Transfer this fragment to a vial with 1.5 ml DMEM. Keep on ice.
7. Put the cryo vials in a cooling rack or on ice (absolutely avoid getting water or ice inside the vial!), and add 1.5 ml of cryopreservation medium (4 °C)
8. Put the tissue fragments two by two in the cryo vials. Close the vials.
9. Leave the vials on ice water/cooling element for 15 min.
10. Put the vials in a cooled container with propanodial.

    Transfer the propanodial container to a −80 °C freezer. Leave it there overnight.

11. For sterility control: Collect a fraction of the transport medium, of DMEM of the last washing dish (petridish 3) and of the cryopreservation medium, and put it in tubes for sterility testing.

Next day: Transfer the vials from the −80 °C freezer to the LN2 container. Freeze in the vapour phase in case of screw-cap vials.

References

1. Meng X, Lindahl M, Hyvönen ME et al (2000) Regulation of cell fate decision of undifferentiated spermatogonia by GDNF. Science 287:1489–1493
2. Song HW, Wilkinson MF (2014) Transcriptional control of spermatogonial maintenance and differentiation. Semin Cell Dev Biol 30:14–26
3. Buaas FW, Kirsh AL, Sharma M et al (2004) Plzf is required in adult male germ cells for stem cell self-renewal. Nat Genet 36:647–652
4. Costoya JA, Hobbs RM, Barna M et al (2004) Essential role of Plzf in maintenance of spermatogonial stem cells. Nat Genet 36:653–659
5. Krausz C, Forti G (2006) Sperm cryopreservation in male infertility due to genetic disorders. Cell Tissue Bank 7:105–112
6. Dakouane M, Albert M, Bergère M et al (2005) Aging and spermatogenesis: an histologic, cytogenetic and apoptosis study. Gynecol Obstet Fertil 33:659–664
7. Meistrich ML (2013) Effects of chemotherapy and radiotherapy on spermatogenesis in humans. Fertil Steril 100:1180–1186
8. Tournaye H, Dohle GR, Barratt CL (2014) Fertility preservation in men with cancer. Lancet 384:1295–1301
9. Nangia AK, Krieg SA, Kim SS (2013) Clinical guidelines for sperm cryopreservation in cancer patients. Fertil Steril 100:1203–1209
10. Lass A, Akagbosu F, Abusheikha N et al (1998) A programme of semen cryopreservation for patients with malignant disease in a tertiary infertility centre: lessons from 8 years' experience. Hum Reprod 13:3256–3261
11. Baniel J, Sella A (2001) Sperm extraction at orchiectomy for testis cancer. Fertil Steril 75:260–262
12. Rosenlund B, Sjöblom P, Törnblom M et al (1998) In-vitro fertilization and intracytoplasmic sperm injection in the treatment of infertility after testicular cancer. Hum Reprod 13:414–418
13. Haddad N, Al-Rabeeah K, Onerheim R, Zini A (2014) Is ex vivo microdissection testicular sperm extraction indicated for infertile men undergoing radical orchiectomy for testicular cancer? Case report and literature review. Fertil Steril 101:956–959
14. Schrader M, Müller M, Sofikitis N et al (2003) Onco-tese: testicular sperm extraction in azoospermic cancer patients before chemotherapy-new guidelines? Urology 61:421–425
15. Berookhim BM, Mulhall JP (2014) Outcomes of operative sperm retrieval strategies for fertility preservation among males scheduled to undergo cancer treatment. Fertil Steril 101:801–811
16. Avarbock MR, Brinster CJ, Brinster RL (1996) Reconstitution of spermatogenesis from frozen spermatogonial stem cells. Nat Med 2:693–696
17. McCook A (2013) A future, on ice. Nat Med 19:958–961
18. Brinster RL, Zimmerman JW (1994) Spermatogenesis following germ cell transplantation. Proc Natl Acad Sci U S A 91:11298–11302
19. Shinohara T, Inoue K, Ogonuki N et al (2002) Birth of offspring following transplantation of cryopreserved immature testicular pieces and in-vitro microinsemination. Hum Reprod 17:3039–3045

20. Hermann BP, Sukhwani M, Winkler F et al (2012) Spermatogonial stem cell transplantation into rhesus testes regenerates spermatogenesis producing functional sperm. Cell Stem Cell 11:715–726
21. Keros V, Hultenby K, Borgström B et al (2007) Methods of cryopreservation of testicular tissue with viable spermatogonia in pre-pubertal boys undergoing gonadotoxic cancer treatment. Hum Reprod 22:1384–1395
22. Curaba M, Poels J, van Langendonckt A et al (2011) Can prepubertal human testicular tissue be cryopreserved by vitrification? Fertil Steril 95:2123.e9–2123.e12
23. Baert Y, Van Saen D, Haentjens P et al (2013) What is the best cryopreservation protocol for human testicular tissue banking? Hum Reprod 28:1816–1826
24. Kanatsu-Shinohara M, Ogonuki N, Iwano T et al (2005) Genetic and epigenetic properties of mouse male germline stem cells during long-term culture. Development 132:4155–4163
25. Sadri-Ardekani H, Mizrak SC, van Daalen SK et al (2009) Propagation of human spermatogonial stem cells in vitro. JAMA 302:2127–2134
26. Sadri-Ardekani H, Akhondi MA, van der Veen F et al (2011) In vitro propagation of human prepubertal spermatogonial stem cells. JAMA 305:2416–2418
27. Nickkholgh B, Mizrak SC, van Daalen SK et al (2014) Genetic and epigenetic stability of human spermatogonial stem cells during long-term culture. Fertil Steril 102:1700–1707
28. Eildermann K, Gromoll J, Behr R (2012) Misleading and reliable markers to differentiate between primate testis-derived multipotent stromal cells and spermatogonia in culture. Hum Reprod 27:1754–1767
29. Kossack N, Terwort N, Wistuba J, Ehmcke J, Schlatt S, Schöler H, Kliesch S, Gromoll J (2013) A combined approach facilitates the reliable detection of human spermatogonia in vitro. Hum Reprod 28:3012–3025
30. Zheng Y, Thomas A, Schmidt CM, Dann CT (2014) Quantitative detection of human spermatogonia for optimization of spermatogonial stem cell culture. Hum Reprod 29:2497–2511
31. Baert Y, Braye A, Struijk RB, van Pelt AMM, Goossens E (2015) Comparable testicular cell dynamics in long-term cultures derived from either fresh or cryopreserved tissues. Fertil Steril 104(5):1244–1252
32. Goossens E, De Rycke M, Haentjens P, Tournaye H (2009) DNA methylation patterns of spermatozoa and two generations of offspring obtained after murine spermatogonial stem cell transplantation. Hum Reprod 24:2255–2263
33. Goossens E, Bilgec T, Van Saen D, Tournaye H (2011) Mouse germ cells go through typical epigenetic modifications after intratesticular tissue grafting. Hum Reprod 26:3388–3400
34. de Vos Goossens E, Tournaye H (2010) Array comparative genomic hybridization analysis does not show genetic alterations in spermatozoa and offspring generated after spermatogonial stem cell transplantation in the mouse. Hum Reprod 25:1836–1842
35. Jahnukainen K, Hou M, Petersen C et al (2001) Intratesticular transplantation of testicular cells from leukemic rats causes transmission of leukemia. Cancer Res 61:706–710
36. Dovey SL, Valli H, Hermann BP et al (2013) Eliminating malignant contamination from therapeutic human spermatogonial stem cells. J Clin Invest 123:1833–1843
37. Sadri-Ardekani H, Homburg CH, van Capel TM et al (2014) Eliminating acute lymphoblastic leukemia cells from human testicular cell cultures: a pilot study. Fertil Steril 101:1072–1078
38. van den Berg H, Repping S, van der Veen F (2007) Parental desire and acceptability of spermatogonial stem cell cryopreservation in boys with cancer. Hum Reprod 22:594–597
39. Sadri-Ardekani H, Akhondi MM, Vossough P et al (2013) Parental attitudes towards fertility preservation in boys with cancer: context of different risk levels of infertility and success rates of fertility restoration. Fertil Steril 99:796–802
40. Wyns C, Curaba M, Petit S et al (2011) Management of fertility preservation in prepubertal patients: 5 years' experience at the Catholic University of Louvain. Hum Reprod 26:737–747
41. Ginsberg JP, Li Y, Carlson CA (2014) Testicular tissue cryopreservation in prepubertal male children: an analysis of parental decision-making. Pediatr Blood Cancer 61:1673–1678

Chapter 10
IVA and Ovarian Tissue Cryopreservation

Kazuhiro Kawamura

Abstract Ovarian primordial follicles do not regenerate and proliferate in vivo, and their number decreases with aging as well as with certain pathogeneses. When the number of residual follicles decreases to a threshold level, the initial step of follicle development, namely, the activation of dormant follicles, is disturbed and subsequent follicle growth is suppressed resulting in anovulation and amenorrhea with high gonadotropin levels. If the amenorrhea occurs before 40 years of age, these patients are diagnosed as primary ovarian insufficiency (POI). POI patients show infertility and symptoms caused by estrogen deficiency. So far, donor egg is an only option for effective infertility treatment in patients with POI; we sought to develop a new approach for infertility treatment using their own eggs. Although POI patients still have dormant residual follicles, they are resistant to endogenous signals for activation. Thus, we attempted to activate the residual follicles in vitro. Because the exact mechanisms of the activation of dormant primordial follicles still remain to be determined, we focused on intracellular signaling in the activation process and succeeded in activating those follicles through the activation of PI3K-Akt-Foxo3 pathway (IVA; in vitro activation). Based on the success of IVA, we performed clinical studies to generate mature oocytes from patients with primary ovarian insufficiency, who had few residual follicles in their ovaries, and we have reported successful pregnancies and a birth following IVA. In this chapter, I show our IVA approach and discuss future possibilities for the infertility treatment in patients with diminished ovarian reserve.

Keywords In vitro activation • Primary ovarian insufficiency • Infertility treatment • Akt signal • Hippo signal

---

K. Kawamura (✉)
Department of Obstetrics and Gynecology, St. Marianna University School of Medicine, 2-16-1 Sugao, Miyamae-ku, Kawasaki, Kanagawa 216-8511, Japan
e-mail: kazuhironanami@gmail.com

N. Suzuki, J. Donnez (eds.), *Gonadal Tissue Cryopreservation in Fertility Preservation*, DOI 10.1007/978-4-431-55963-4_10

10.1 Introduction

The ovaries have primordial follicles that grow into eggs. The number of primordial follicles, which reaches its peak during fetal life, does not increase after birth but decreases with aging. Around puberty, the ovary has several hundred thousand primordial follicles, which generally remain dormant. After the first menstruation, as many as 1,000 dormant primordial follicles per month are activated for initiation of growth. They receive the paracrine and endocrine effects of the factors produced locally in the ovary and gonadotropins secreted by the pituitary gland, respectively, and continue to grow. A primordial follicle matures into a primary follicle, secondary follicle (pre-antral follicle, antral follicle), and preovulatory follicle, and then ovulation occurs. When the number of residual primordial follicles in the ovary decreases to less than 1,000, the regular activation of follicles no longer occurs, and recruitment of developing follicles stops. As the result, estrogen, which is secreted by the granulosa cells of grown follicles, then declines, leading to cause menopause symptoms and amenorrhea due to the insufficient proliferation of the endometrium. At the same time, ovulation arrests and menstruation stops [1].

Primary ovarian insufficiency (POI) is a disease in which the follicles in the ovaries rapidly decrease and the number of remaining follicles falls below the threshold (≦about 1,000) in women younger than 40 years. Thus, POI is sometimes referred to as premature ovarian failure. POI is not a rare disease because 1 in every 100 women spontaneously develops it [2]. The various causes of POI—chromosomal abnormality, gene abnormality, autoimmune disease, and iatrogenic factors (ovarian surgery, chemotherapy, and radiotherapy)—have been identified. However, there are many cases of POI for which the cause is unknown [3, 4]. Because POI patients show arrest of spontaneous ovulation at early age resulting in loss of their fertility, they are totally resistant to infertility treatment. To date, the most effective infertility treatments for POI patients to become pregnant are in vitro fertilization and embryo transfer (IVF-ET) using donor eggs from young women. Generally, these patients unlikely become pregnant with their own eggs. However, IVF-ET with donor eggs is not allowed all over the world. Most women would prefer to become pregnant not with donor eggs but with their own eggs. In a case of Japan where the highest number of IVF-ET program is conducted in the world, although egg donation is not prohibited in Japan, in principle, the view is that eggs should be donated for free from young women and donors are asked to receive invasive interventions, such as ovarian stimulations and oocyte retrievals. In light of this, the number of egg donors is extremely limited in Japan. Thus, Japanese patients in need of donor eggs usually seek fertility treatment with donor eggs in foreign countries.

In this chapter, we introduce detail techniques for the in vitro activation (IVA) of dormant primordial follicles that we have developed and report on the status of the ongoing clinical application of IVA, along with its future prospect.

10.2 Follicle Growth

The follicular growth from primordial to preovulatory stages is classified into three phases, according to their gonadotropin dependence (Fig. 10.1) [5]. In the first phase, in which primordial follicles become pre-natral follicles, follicles at these stages develop in a gonadotropin-independent manner. The meiosis of oocytes that reach the diplotene stage of the prophase of meiotic division before birth is arrested at the state of primordial follicles, and the primordial follicles become dormant until pubertal. When the menstrual cycle is established after birth, some primordial follicles initiate to develop following the menstrual cycle. In general, primordial follicles are activated at the rate of ~1,000 follicles/cycle and become primary follicles. However, the precise mechanism for the selection of dormant primordial follicles to be activated from the many primordial follicles has not been determined [1].

The second phase of follicular development, from a pre-antral follicle to an antral follicle of less than 2 mm in diameter, is called as the gonadotropin-responsive phase. In this phase, a follicle is not affected by changes in the gonadotropins associated with the menstrual cycle, but develops depending on the stimulation by basal gonadotropins. When antral follicles of more than 2 mm in diameter reach the gonadotropin-dependent phase, they rapidly increase due to the increase in gonadotropins associated with the menstrual cycle and develop into preovulatory follicles.

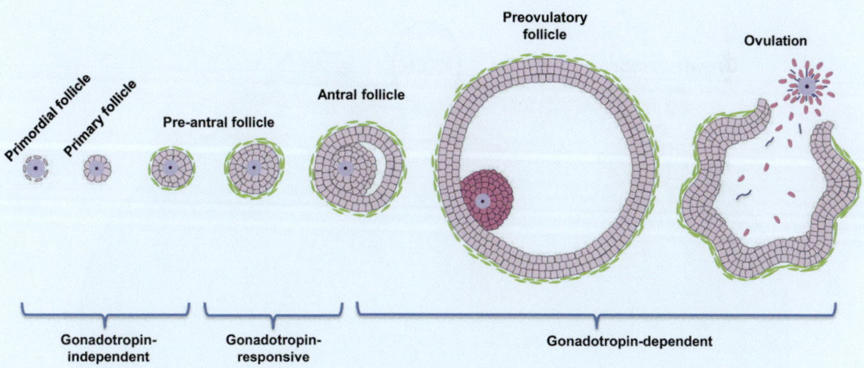

Fig. 10.1 Human follicle development and its dependence on gonadotropins

10.3 Artificial Activation of Dormant Primordial Follicles, IVA (In Vitro Activation)

Recently, our research team and another group demonstrated that as the mechanism is involved in the control of the activation of dormant primordial follicles, the phosphoinositide 3-kinase (PI3K)-Akt-Forkhead box O3 (FOXO3) signal pathway induced the activation of follicles (Fig. 10.2). FOXO3 acts to arrest the cell cycle in the nuclei and controls the activation of primordial follicles. If the PI3K-Akt signal turns on in the dormant follicles, FOXO3 is transferred from the nucleus to cytoplasm and loses its function, resulting in activation of dormant primordial follicles. In the ovaries, primordial follicles are dormant and not activated because phosphatase with tensin homolog deleted in chromosome 10 (PTEN) inhibits the PI3K-Akt signaling pathway. Among many dormant primordial follicles, some follicles are selected to be activated by unknown mechanisms. The selected follicles are activated by some signals that may release the PI3K-Akt signaling pathway inhibited by PTEN or that may exceed the inhibitory effect of PTEN. Then, FOXO3 is transferred from the nucleus to cytoplasm, and some dormant primordial follicles start to grow.

These mechanisms for regulation of the activation of dormant primordial follicles have been clarified by a series of studies based on phenotyping of the ovaries of PTEN and FOXO3 gene-deficient mice [6–9], the culture of mouse/human ovarian tissues with a PTEN inhibitor and PI3K activator, and transplantation of mouse/human ovaries that had been subjected to the activation of dormant primordial follicles by treatment with the use of a PTEN inhibitor and PI3K activator into a

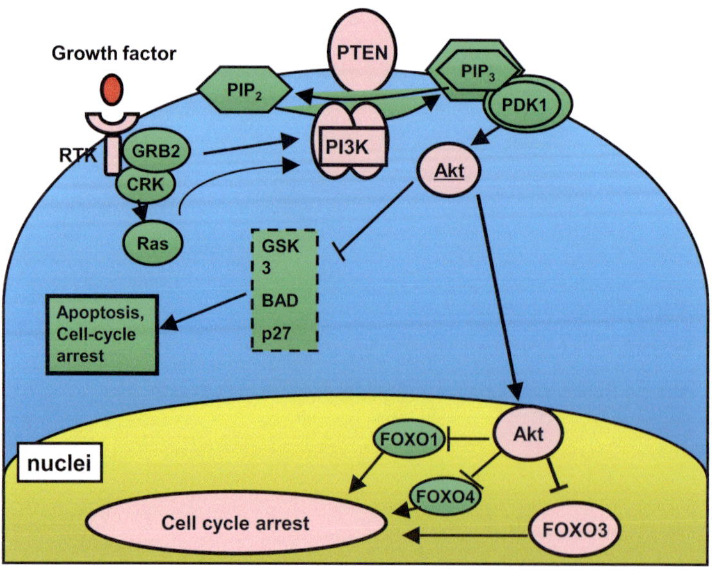

Fig. 10.2 Activation of dormant primordial follicles through PTEN-PI3K-Akt-Foxo3 signaling pathway

mouse [8]. In an ovum-specific, conditional PTEN-deficient mouse, the primordial follicles in the ovary are activated spontaneously, and follicular growth begins, resulting in enlarged ovaries with multiple growing follicles. The pool of primordial follicles in the ovary is depleted at an early stage of life, and no follicles are observed in the ovary of a 16-week-old female mouse. The phenotype observed in this mouse is close to that observed in a patient with POI [6–8]. In FOXO3-deficient mice, the spontaneous activation of dormant primordial follicles and subsequent phenotype similar to that observed in POI were also reported [9].

A 3-day-old female mouse has only primordial follicles in its ovaries. After the transient treatment of the ovary with a PTEN inhibitor and PI3K activator, as in the case of the PTEN gene-deficient mice, the primordial follicles were activated and started to grow [10]. In human, we obtained normal parts of the ovary from patients with a benign ovarian tumor and prepared ovarian fragments for in vitro cultures. After the transient treatment of these fragments with a PTEN inhibitor, activation of the primordial follicles was detected [10]. Furthermore, the ovaries of 3-day-old mice were treated with a PTEN inhibitor and PI3K activator to activate dormant primordial follicles in vitro. The murine ovaries were transplanted under the kidney capsule of adult mice that had undergone ovarian resection to increase endogenous gonadotropins. Then, FSH was administrated to the animals to stimulate growth of activated follicles. Eighteen days after transplantation, the primordial follicles developed into preovulatory stage, and mature oocytes were obtained from the transplanted ovaries at 14 after hCG injection. After in vitro fertilization with these mature eggs and embryo transfer to pseudopregnant mice, we found normal pregnancy and delivered pups. Moreover, as demonstrated by methylation analyses of Igf2r, Litl, and H19 genes, the mature eggs obtained using this method had normal genome imprinting and showed no abnormality of the structures, including the spindle apparatus [10]. In the next experiment with the above-referenced human ovarian fragments, the human primordial follicles were treated with a PTEN inhibitor for activation. These ovarian fragments were transplanted under the kidney capsule of severe combined immunodeficiency (SCID) mice that had undergone ovarian resection to increase endogenous gonadotropins. Because it takes 6 months for human primordial follicles to develop to preovulatory stage, the transplanted ovarian fragments were dissected from the SCID mice after 6 months of grafting, and the follicular growth was examined by histological analyses. We found many large antral follicles developed in the ovarian fragments and obtained mature human eggs from those follicles [10]. Eventually, we named this approach for in vitro activation of follicles to be "IVA (in vitro activation)."

10.4 Clinical Application of IVA

A diagnosis of POI is made if a woman less than 40 years of age presents with hypergonadotropic amenorrhea. This is a condition characterized by the absence of growing follicles in the ovary. A patient with POI is infertile because of disruption of ovarian functions leading lack of ovulation. Although a wide variety of causes, including chromosomal abnormality, autoimmune disease, and iatrogenic factors, are involved in the development of POI, as a common pathological condition, the rapid decrease of follicles remaining in the ovary has been pointed out. If the number of residual primordial follicles declines to the menopausal level and falls to approximately 1,000, their activation rarely occurs, follicle recruitment stops, and the growing follicles disappear [1]. Thus, patients present with serious treatment-resistant infertility because ovulation does not occur. To date, the most effective treatment for patients with POI who wish to become pregnant is IVF-ET using donated eggs. However, the donor egg program is limited to be available in some countries including Southeast Asia and the United States. One in every 100 women spontaneously is known to develop POI. Although not all patients with POI wish to bear children, there is a definite shortage of donated eggs in the worlds. In some countries, the recent trend toward delayed marriage increases number of infertile POI patients, because POI patients can become pregnant and bear children before the development of POI completely.

Conventionally, various hormone therapies and ovulation induction treatments have been prescribed for patients who have few residual follicles in their ovaries. Because these treatments have a limited effect, the development of a new method for treating infertility that would enable patients to become pregnant using their own eggs has been much anticipated. We conducted animal experiments to confirm the safety of IVA. We then clinically applied this technique followed by IVF-ET for the first time ever in POI patients with approval from the ethical committee and consent from the patients (Fig. 10.3) [11]. Other research groups also examined the safety of this technique and confirmed that it was safe [12]. Our clinical study of IVA is briefly explained below.

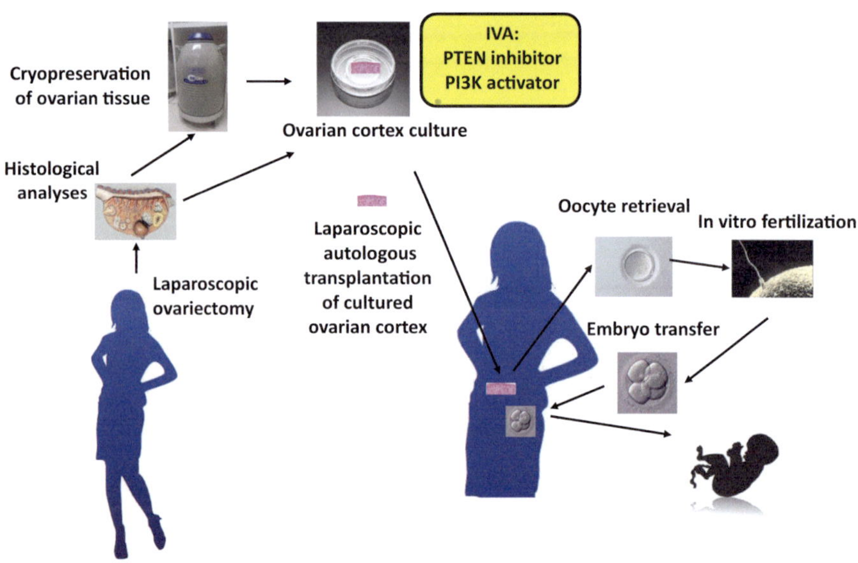

Fig. 10.3 Clinical application of IVA

10.4.1 Laparoscopic Ovariectomy

We performed a laparoscopic ovariectomy to reduce the effects of an invasive treatment on the patients and to minimize postoperative intraperitoneal adhesion in preparation for subsequent ovarian transplantation. In patients with POI, the ovaries frequently can be resected without requiring hemostasis by electrocoagulation because of poor blood flow around the ovaries. Fallopian tubes are used later as sites for ovarian transplantation. Therefore, they must not be damaged by the surgical procedure or affected by electrocoagulation of the ovarian stumps. The surgeon must carefully resect the ovary by itself.

10.4.2 Ovarian Tissue Cryopreservation, Histological Analysis to Detect Residual Ovarian Follicles

From the resected ovaries, the cortex where the follicles are localized is isolated from the medulla and cut into 1 × 1 cm stripes. These ovarian tissues are subjected to the culture for activation of follicles. Part of the ovarian tissue is fixed to prepare the sections. The sections are stained with hematoxylin and eosin (HE) to confirm the presence/absence of residual follicles. We use the vitrification technique for temporary cryopreserve of the ovarian cortex after ovariectomy. Although this cryopreservation process of the ovary is not essential for IVA, it provides several benefits. (1) Because POI is a progressive disease, the number of residual primordial follicles decreases over the course of time. A patient with POI can prepare for future IVA if she undergoes resection of an ovary for cryopreservation immediately after being diagnosed with POI. In this case, the high possibility also exists that follicles may grow incidentally in the remaining ovary at that time. Therefore, we perform hormone therapy and expect ovulation. If follicular growth cannot be observed for some time, the frozen ovarian tissues are thawed for IVA. (2) For IVA, we cannot use all ovarian cortical tissues due to the limitation of transplantation sites beneath serosa of Fallopian tubes as described below. Because the transplanted ovarian fragments are adsorbed and disappear after 1–2 years of grafting, we can repeat transplantation of ovaries with activation of follicles if we cryopreserve the remaining ovarian tissues. Indeed, in patients with POI, the residual follicles are not distributed uniformly in the ovarian cortex. Therefore, the possibility of grafting of small fragments containing the residual follicles increases by repeating the transplantation procedure. (3) Ovarian transplantation must be conducted 2 days after ovariectomy if the ovarian tissues cannot be cryopreserved. The technique of cryopreservation enables us to avoid the repetition of surgeries for a short period of time.

10.4.3 Ovarian Tissue Culture

The thawed ovarian cortices are cut into small cubic or cuboid fragments 1–2 mm in size. The PI3K-Akt signal is activated by a 48 h ovarian tissue culture with a PTEN inhibitor and PI3K activator [11].

10.4.4 Autologous Transplantation of Cultured Ovarian Fragments

After completion of the culture, the ovarian tissues are thoroughly washed, and an autologous transplantation is performed under laparoscopic surgery. Due to the poor blood flow in the ovaries of patients with POI, transplanted ovarian fragments considered to be difficult to survive with neovascularization. Ovary engraftment seems to be difficult. Therefore, we select the site beneath the serosa of the Fallopian tubes for transplantation because this site has sufficient blood flow, can be observed easily by transvaginal ultrasound, and requires no special oocyte retrieval procedure for IVF-ET.

10.4.5 Monitoring Follicle Growth and IVF-ET

After the autologous transplantation of the ovary, hormone tests (LH, FSH, and E2) and a transvaginal ultrasound are conducted to detect follicular growth every 1–2 weeks. When follicular growth is achieved, oocytes are retrieved as the same method of conventional IVF procedures. If mature eggs are obtained, eggs are fertilized by either insemination or ICSI (intracytoplasmic sperm injection) and cultured to develop to preimplantation embryos at early cleavage stage. Then, these embryos are cryopreserved by the vitrification technique. After induction of withdrawal bleeding by hormonal treatments, the thawed embryos are transferred under hormone replacement cycles.

10.4.6 Clinical Outcome of IVA

By the time our first paper was published, we had conducted ovariectomy in 27 patients with POI (mean age 37.3 ± 5.8 years, mean period of amenorrhea 6.8 ± 2.1 years) and, histologically, confirmed residual follicles in 13 of 27 patients. IVA-ovarian transplantation was performed in all the patients with ovariectomy. During the 1-year observation period after transplantation, follicular growth was detected in 8 of 13 patients with residual follicles, and mature eggs were obtained in

5 of 8 patients. Of note, no follicular growth was found in the 14 patients who had no residual follicles in the histological examination during the observation period. By the time the paper was published, we had conducted frozen-thawed embryo transfer in three patients and confirmed that two of them were pregnant. One patient suffered a miscarriage in early pregnancy, while the other had a successful pregnancy. At 37 weeks and 2 days of pregnancy, she delivered a normal boy weighing 3,254 g through a cesarean section because of breech presentation [11].

10.5 Stimulation of Secondary Follicle Growth by Suppression Hippo Signaling Pathway in IVA

In humans, a primordial follicle requires 6 months to develop into a preovulatory follicle [5, 10]. Therefore, we predicted that follicular growth after IVA might occur 6 months after ovarian transplantation. In some of our patients, however, follicles grew within 1 month after transplantation. We hypothesized that this phenomenon occurred because not just primordial follicles but also secondary follicles grew after IVA. We then attempted to clarify the molecular mechanism involved in the phenomenon.

A Hippo signal is an important intracellular signal in controlling cell proliferation and determining organ size. It is inactivated by impaired intercellular adhesion or cytoskeletal change [13–15]. Generally, Yes-associated protein (YAP), an effector protein, is phosphorylated by the Hippo signal, and its transport to the nucleus is prevented. However, by inhibiting the Hippo signal, YAP phosphorylation is canceled, and YAP is transported to the nucleus and coupled with TEAD, a nuclear transcription factor, to promote the production of CCN growth factors for cell proliferation [13, 16]. In IVA, the ovary is cut into small fragments 1–2 mm in size for tissue culture. In this process, the Hippo signal is suppressed, and in turn the granulosa cells proliferate to promote follicular growth. On the basis of this hypothesis, we have conducted a series of studies.

In mouse and human ovaries, all of the Hippo family's genes were expressed in granulosa cells. By cutting the ovary into small fragments, the Hippo signal was suppressed, YAP was transported to the nucleus of the granulosa cell, and CCN growth factors then increased rapidly leading to stimulation of secondary follicle growth. Moreover, we found that, like the process of cutting the ovary into small fragments, the addition of CCN growth factors to the ovarian tissue culture promoted the growth of secondary follicles. The effects of secondary follicle growth by the process of cutting the ovary into small fragments were inhibited by the verteporfin that inhibited the bond between YAP and TEAD and the neutralizing antibodies against for CCN growth factors. It is known that cytoskeletal actin polymerization inhibits the Hippo signal [17, 18]. We demonstrated that cutting the mouse ovary into small fragments resulted in temporary actin polymerization leading to inhibition of the Hippo signal. Thus, we clarified the molecular

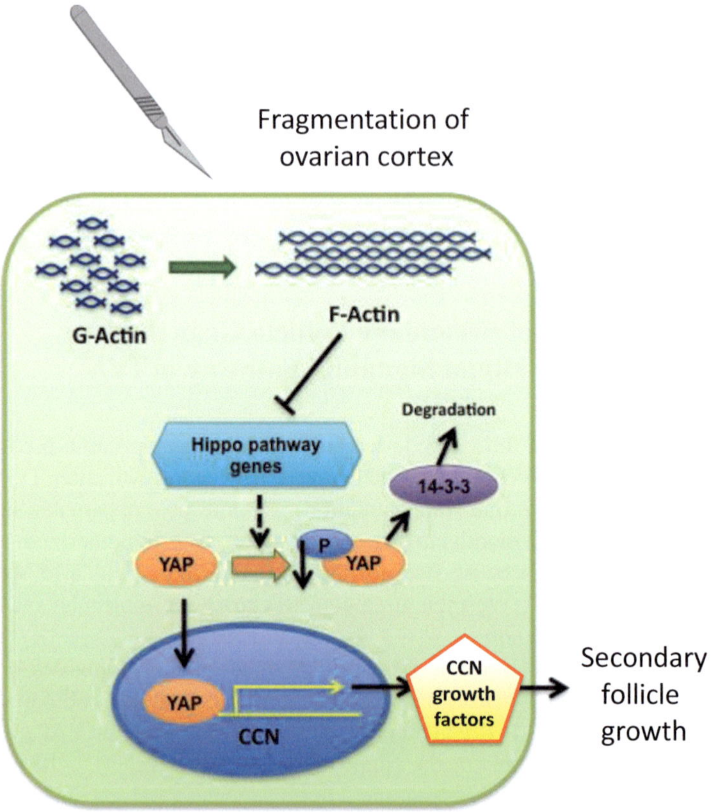

Fig. 10.4 Molecular mechanisms of stimulation of secondary follicle growth by fragmentation of ovaries

mechanism involved in the process from cutting the ovary into small fragments, through actin polymerization, inhibition of the Hippo signal, transfer of YAP to the nucleus, and production of CCN growth factors, to growth of secondary follicles (Fig. 10.4).

10.6 Conclusion and Future Perspective of IVA

We could achieve to develop novel infertility treatment in patients with POI [11, 19, 20]. The IVA approach is effective not only for POI patients but also for patients with poor responder patients with diminishing ovarian reserve including aging patients. In aging patients, it is important to note that IVA treatment has potential to increase number of oocytes retrieved to give a chance to have high quality embryos, but cannot improve the quality of the oocytes. Although we tested the safety of IVA approach for clinical application intensively by animal studies and a healthy baby was born, more studies are needed to ensure the safety of the present IVA procedure.

The IVA approach contains two laparoscopic surgeries. To decrease the invasiveness to the patients, we are now trying to establish a medical treatment to activate follicles without surgeries by direct administration of Akt stimulators and/or Hippo signaling inhibitors [21]. In the POI patients enrolled in this clinical study, only half of patients had residual follicles by histological analyses. The patients without detected follicles by histology did not respond to IVA treatment. However, it is difficult to predict the absence/presence of residual follicles through noninvasive procedures before ovariectomy. Indeed, majority of POI patients showed elevated gonadotropin levels and undetectable anti-Mullerian hormone levels in spite of presence or absence of ovarian follicles [20]. Thus, we are also seeking to identify ultrasensitive markers to be able to evaluate the presence of residua follicles even in the POI patients. Because IVA is only effective in patients with residual follicles, we expect to determine the indication of IVA treatment by establishment of a method for measurement of ultrasensitive biomarkers that indicate more accurate information about the presence of residual follicles than conventional tests.

Acknowledgments This work was supported by Grant-In-Aid for Scientific Research (Challenging Exploratory Research: 15K15613, and Innovative Areas, Mechanisms regulating gamete formation in animals: 26114510) and by research funds from the Grant for Fertility Innovation, the Smoking Research Foundation, and the Takeda Science Foundation. None of the authors has a conflict of interest.

References

1. Macklon NS, Fauser BC (1999) Aspects of ovarian follicle development throughout life. Horm Res 52:161–170. doi:10.1159/000023456
2. Coulam CB, Stringfellow S, Hoefnagel D (1983) Evidence for a genetic factor in the etiology of premature ovarian failure. Fertil Steril 40:693–695
3. Nelson LM (2009) Clinical practice. Primary ovarian insufficiency. N Engl J Med 360:606–614. doi:10.1056/NEJMcp0808697
4. De Vos M, Devroey P, Fauser BC (2010) Primary ovarian insufficiency. Lancet 376:911–921. doi:10.1016/S0140-6736(10)60355-8
5. McGee EA, Hsueh AJ (2000) Initial and cyclic recruitment of ovarian follicles. Endocr Rev 21:200–214. doi:10.1210/edrv.21.2.0394
6. Reddy P, Liu L, Adhikari D et al (2008) Oocyte-specific deletion of Pten causes premature activation of the primordial follicle pool. Science 319:611–613. doi:10.1126/science.1152257
7. John GB, Gallardo TD, Shirley LJ, Castrillon DH (2008) Foxo3 is a PI3K-dependent molecular switch controlling the initiation of oocyte growth. Dev Biol 321:197–204. doi:10.1016/j-ydbio.2008.06.017
8. Adhikari D, Liu K (2009) Molecular mechanisms underlying the activation of mammalian primordial follicles. Endocr Rev 30:438–464. doi:10.1210/er.2008-0048

9. Castrillon DH, Miao L, Kollipara R et al (2003) Suppression of ovarian follicle activation in mice by the transcription factor Foxo3a. Science 301:215–218. doi:10.1126/science.1086336
10. Li J, Kawamura K, Cheng Y et al (2010) Activation of dormant ovarian follicles to generate mature eggs. Proc Natl Acad Sci U S A 107:10280–10284. doi:10.1073/pnas.1001198107
11. Kawamura K, Cheng Y, Suzuki N et al (2013) Hippo signaling disruption and Akt stimulation of ovarian follicles for infertility treatment. Proc Natl Acad Sci U S A 110:17474–17479. doi:10.1073/pnas.1312830110
12. Adhikari D, Gorre N, Risal S et al (2012) The safe use of a PTEN inhibitor for the activation of dormant mouse primordial follicles and generation of fertilizable eggs. PLoS One 7:e39034. doi:10.1371/jounal.pone.0039034
13. Pan D (2007) Hippo signaling in organ size control. Genes Dev 21:886–897. doi:10.1101/gad.1536007
14. Halder G, Johnson RL (2011) Hippo signaling: growth control and beyond. Development 138:9–22. doi:10.1242/dev.045500
15. Hergovich A (2012) Mammalian Hippo signalling: a kinase network regulated by proteinprotein interactions. Biochem Soc Trans 40:124–128. doi:10.1042/BST20110619
16. Holbourn KP, Acharya KR, Perbal B (2008) The CCN family of proteins: structure-function relationships. Trends Biochem Sci 33:461–473. doi:10.1016/j.tibs.2008.07.006
17. Sansores Garcia L, Bossuyt W, Wada K et al (2012) Modulating F-actin organization induces organ growth by affecting the Hippo pathway. EMBO J 30:2325–2335. doi:10.1038/emboj.2011.157
18. Fernandez BG, Gasoar P, Bras Pereira C et al (2012) Actin-capping protein and the Hippo pathway regulate F-actin and tissue growth in drosophila. Development 138:2337–2346. doi:10.1242/dev.063545
19. Hsueh AJ, Kawamura K, Cheng Y, Fauser BC (2015) Intraovarian control of early folliculogenesis. Endocr Rev 36(1):1–24. doi:10.1210/er.2014-1020
20. Suzuki N, Yoshioka N, Takae S et al (2015) Successful fertility preservation following ovarian tissue vitrification in patients with primary ovarian insufficiency. Hum Reprod 30(3):608–615. doi:10.1093/humrep/deu353
21. Cheng Y, Feng Y, Jansson L et al (2015) Actin polymerization-enhancing drugs promote ovarian follicle growth mediated by the Hippo signaling effector YAP. FASEB J 29 (6):2423–2430. doi:10.1096/fj.14-267856

Chapter 11
Risk of Transferring Malignant Cells with Transplanted Frozen-Thawed Ovarian Tissue

Marie-Madeleine Dolmans and Michelle Soares

Abstract Although ovarian tissue cryopreservation and transplantation have emerged as a real option to preserve and restore fertility in young cancer patients, there is a legitimate concern regarding the possible presence of malignant cells in the ovarian tissue, which could lead to recurrence of the disease after reimplantation. The present chapter reviews the existing literature on the subject to evaluate the risk of transplanting malignant cells in case of the main malignant indications for ovarian tissue cryopreservation.

Keywords Ovarian tissue cryopreservation • Ovarian tissue transplantation • Cancer • Risks • Malignant cells

11.1 Introduction

In women who require cancer treatment but cannot delay the start of chemotherapy, as well as prepubertal patients, cryopreservation of ovarian tissue is the main, and sometimes the only, fertility preservation option available [1–3].

In the near future, more and more cancer patients cured of their disease will request reimplantation of their cryopreserved ovarian tissue. However, there is a concern regarding the possible presence of malignant cells in the ovarian tissue, which could lead to recurrence of the primary disease after reimplantation [4].

In our department, hematological malignancies are the most common indication for ovarian tissue cryopreservation, representing 37.5 % of all indications [5].

M.-M. Dolmans (✉)
Pôle de Recherche en Gynécologie, Institut de Recherche Expérimentale et Clinique (IREC), Cliniques Universitaires Saint Luc, Avenue Mounier 52, B1.52.02, 1200 Brussels, Belgium

Département de Gynécologie, Cliniques Universitaires Saint-Luc, 1200 Brussels, Belgium
e-mail: marie-madeleine.dolmans@uclouvain.be

M. Soares
Pôle de Recherche en Gynécologie, Institut de Recherche Expérimentale et Clinique (IREC), Cliniques Universitaires Saint Luc, Avenue Mounier 52, B1.52.02, 1200 Brussels, Belgium

N. Suzuki, J. Donnez (eds.), *Gonadal Tissue Cryopreservation in Fertility Preservation*, DOI 10.1007/978-4-431-55963-4_11

In this category, Hodgkin's lymphoma (HL) is the most frequent, followed by leukemia and then non-Hodgkin's lymphoma (NHL). According to the literature (SEER), the most common hematological cancer in females under the age of 20 is leukemia, followed by HL and then NHL.

The aim of this chapter is to examine all available evidence of the risks of transplanting malignant cells with frozen-thawed ovarian tissue from cancer patients. These risks are evaluated for each of the main indications for ovarian tissue cryopreservation.

11.2 Leukemia

Meirow et al. [6] were the first to detect malignant cells in frozen-thawed ovarian tissue from a patient with chronic myeloid leukemia (CML) by real-time quantitative polymerase chain reaction (RT-qPCR). A retrospective analysis of 5571 autopsy findings of females under the age of 40 in Japan also found, by histology, leukemic involvement of the ovaries in 8.4 % of leukemia patients [7].

In recent studies, molecular biology was used to evaluate the presence of leukemic cells in cryopreserved ovarian tissue from patients with CML, acute myeloid leukemia (AML), and acute lymphoblastic leukemia (ALL), leukemia types that are the most frequent indications for cryopreservation of ovarian tissue [8–12].

11.2.1 Detection of Malignant Cells in Cryopreserved Ovarian Tissue from Patients with Leukemia

11.2.1.1 Ovarian Tissue Histology

Although in the abovementioned studies [8, 9], histology and immunohistochemistry failed to detect malignant cells in fresh or frozen ovarian tissue from any leukemia patients, we should stress that since these publications, malignant cells have been detected by histology/immunohistochemistry in three cases of ALL [4].

11.2.1.2 Determination of BCR-ABL Fusion Gene Transcripts (PCR Analysis)

The Philadelphia chromosome is pathognomonic for CML, and specific breakpoint cluster region/proto-oncogene tyrosine protein kinase ABL1 (BCR–ABL1) transcripts can be identified using RT-qPCR [3, 13]. Other specific translocations (e.g., t[1;19]) may be present in ALL disease. In disseminated residual disease (MDD) studies, PCR analysis was performed on blood and bone marrow at the time of diagnosis, and the same markers were used on frozen-thawed ovarian tissue.

11.2.1.3 Detection of Clonal Immunoglobulin and T-Cell Receptor Gene Recombinations (PCR Analysis)

RT-qPCR analysis of leukemia-specific junctional regions of rearranged immunoglobulin (Ig) genes and T-cell receptor (TCR) genes was also performed in case of ALL. Occasionally, no chromosomal abnormalities are evidenced in ALL patients, but specific immunoglobulin gene rearrangements can often be tested, even if the sensitivity of these assays is lower. It should be noted that some ALL cases do not display any markers at all, so the risk of contamination by malignant cells cannot be evaluated by PCR in these cases.

11.2.2 Is There a Risk of Malignant Cell Contamination When Ovarian Tissue Is Retrieved from Patients with Leukemia in the Active Phase? [4, 8, 12] (Table 11.1)

Molecular detection of leukemic cells in ovarian tissue can always be carried out for CML, as the presence of the BCR-ABL gene is characteristic of the disease. On the contrary, for ALL, genetic markers are not always detected. Chromosome translocations are reported in almost 50 % of ALL patients. If no chromosomal abnormalities are in blood or bone marrow of ALL patients, specific immunoglobulin gene rearrangements can be investigated, despite the lower sensitivity of these tests (10^{-2}), as stated above.

Among CML patients ($n = 6$), two were found to be positive for the BCR-ABL leukemic marker in their ovarian tissue (Table 11.1). In our series [8], all CML patients underwent ovarian tissue cryopreservation before *sterilizing* chemotherapy, but after receiving hydroxycarbamide, with or without imatinib. We should nevertheless point out that even after a minimum of 6 months of hydroxycarbamide, PCR results showed that ovarian tissue was still positive in two patients.

Among ALL patients ($n = 12$), two were excluded from PCR analysis because no molecular markers were available. Of the remaining ten, seven showed positive molecular markers in their cryopreserved ovarian tissue.

Of the 7 patients who exhibited positive ALL markers, 4 had not received any chemotherapy before ovarian tissue cryopreservation (patients 8, 11, 13, and 14), while 3 had already undergone one regimen of chemotherapy (patients 7, 10, and 18). In case of ALL, gonadotoxic chemotherapy is often initiated before fertility preservation options can be proposed because of the urgency of treatment. It is thus important to establish whether previous chemotherapy can help eliminate malignant cells from ovarian tissue.

In the study published in Blood [8], among the 10 ALL patients with available molecular markers, four women who underwent ovarian tissue cryopreservation

Table 11.1 Patients and pathology characteristics with PCR markers tested on frozen-thawed ovarian tissue

Patient #	Age at OTC	Pathology	gonadotoxic chemotherapy before OTC	Molecular markers	PCR results in ovarian tissue
1	31	CML	0	t(9;22) (q34;q11.2); BCR-ABL	Positive
2	17	CML	0	t(9;22) (q34;q11,2); BCR-ABL	Negative
3	30	CML	0	t(9;22) (q34;q11.2); BCR-ABL	Positive
4	19	CML	0	t(9;22) (q34;q11,2); BCR-ABL	Negative
5	32	CML	0	t(9;22) (q34;q11,2); BCR-ABL	Negative
6	19	CML	0	t(9;22) (q34;q11,2); BCR-ABL	Negative
7	15	ALL	1 (1,8)	t(9;22) (q34;q11.2); BCR-ABL	Positive
8	21	ALL	0	t(1;19) (q23;p13.3); E2A-PBX1	Positive
9	27	ALL	2 (2, 3, 4, 5, 6)	Ig and TCRγ rearrangement genes	Negative
10	20	ALL	1 (1, 2, 3, 4, 7, 8)	Ig and TCRγ rearrangement genes	Positive
11	12	ALL	0	Ig rearrangement genes	Positive
12	15	ALL	1 (1,2)	No molecular marker found	NA
13	15	ALL	0	Ig rearrangement genes	Positive
14	14	ALL	0	Ig rearrangement genes	Positive
15	16	ALL	1 (1,2)	Ig rearrangement genes	Negative
16	5	ALL	1 (1, 2)	Ig and TCRγ rearrangement genes	Negative
17	3	ALL	1 (1,2)	No molecular marker found	NA
18	11	ALL	1 (1, 2)	TCRγ rearrangement genes	Positive

Table showing the number of CML and ALL patients, their age at the time of ovarian tissue cryopreservation (OTC), and the type of gonadotoxic chemotherapy received before OTC (CML patients received hydroxycarbamide with or without imatinib). Molecular markers present in blood or bone marrow at the time of diagnosis were tested by PCR on frozen-thawed ovarian tissue Adapted from Dolmans et al. [8]

Legend: *OTC* ovarian tissue cryopreservation, *Ig* immunoglobulin rearrangement genes, *TCR* T-cell receptor rearrangement genes, *NA* not applicable, *1* methotrexate, *2* cortisone, *3* cyclophosphamide, *4* vincristine, *5* doxorubicin, *6* cytosine arabinoside, *7* daunorubicin, *8* asparaginase

before receiving any chemotherapy showed positive PCR results for the presence of leukemic markers in their ovarian tissue (patients 8, 11, 13, and 14). The remaining six ALL patients with available molecular markers had already received some chemotherapy prior to ovarian tissue cryopreservation. Despite these first regimens of chemotherapy, three patients still exhibited positive ovarian tissue (patients 7, 10, and 18). Moreover, one of them (patient 10) had already received a full cycle of six chemotherapeutic agents (cortisone, methotrexate, cyclophosphamide, vincristine, daunorubicin, and asparaginase). These results indicate that one cycle of chemotherapy is clearly insufficient to completely eliminate all leukemic cells.

We can conclude that by using disease-specific PCR techniques, contamination of ovarian tissue was detected in respectively 33 % and 70 % of CML and ALL patients [8].

11.2.3 Is the Risk Diminished if Ovarian Tissue Is Taken from Patients in Complete Remission? [11]

At the time of diagnosis, a patient with leukemia has a huge number of circulating malignant cells. However, the first or first few rounds of chemotherapy (induction therapy) usually eliminate most of these malignant cells from the blood stream and bone marrow, and the patient enters morphological remission. Nevertheless, malignant cells may persist, even if undetectable, and consolidation therapy is then needed. A subgroup of patients will require allogeneic hematopoietic stem cell transplantation (HSCT) in order to be cured.

Greve et al. evaluated the risk of malignant cell contamination of cryopreserved ovarian cortex from patients with leukemia and found that even in patients in complete remission, traces of malignant cell contamination could be detected by RT-qPCR in two out of four patients with a known molecular marker [11].

Jahnukainen et al. examined ovarian tissue originating from girls who had died from leukemia [13], some in the active phase and some in complete remission. RT-qPCR of ovarian cortex from all patients in the active phase demonstrated the presence of malignant cells, but even in two of the ten patients in remission, traces of malignant cells were still detected, albeit at low levels.

However, to what extent this translates into a real risk of introducing viable malignant cells into patients undergoing transplantation is currently not known with any certainty [12].

Greve et al. transplanted ovarian cortex from 17 patients with ALL or AML to immunodeficient mice. All the women were in complete remission when the ovarian tissue was collected and cryopreserved [11]. None of the mice developed leukemia, indicating that too few copies of malignant cells were present to transmit the disease to mice. What the implication of this result is for humans is less certain, as mice models could well underestimate the real risk because of a lack of species-specific growth factors, or overestimate the risk due to a lack of protection from the immune system of the mouse [12].

11.2.4 In Conclusion

1. The risk of finding viable malignant cells in cryopreserved ovarian tissue from leukemia patients in complete remission is low. However, it cannot be completely excluded [12]. The study by Greve et al. [11] needs to be confirmed by other teams before transplantation can be contemplated in these patients. Furthermore, each type of leukemia may represent a different risk scenario depending on how induction is performed, how far into remission the patient is, and other factors, like the number of viable malignant cells that can cause relapse.
2. New and possibly lifelong treatment with imatinib can remove malignant cells, so they cannot be detected either by blood count (complete hematologic response), cytogenetic detection of the Philadelphia chromosome (complete cytogenetic response), or RT-qPCR (complete molecular remission). However, if patients stop treatment with imatinib, some will relapse [14–16]. While imatinib probably does not pose a threat to fertility [15], it is known to be teratogenic [16]. Patients treated solely with tyrosine kinase inhibitors should not be offered cryopreservation of ovarian tissue, as the treatment is unlikely to cause ovarian insufficiency. Only patients with CML who cannot be brought into complete remission (chronic phase with detectable disease in blood and bone marrow) will need to undergo HSCT and are thus candidates for ovarian tissue cryopreservation [17].

11.3 Lymphoma

Caution should be exercised in case of HL and NHL, which are frequent indications for ovarian tissue cryopreservation [5, 17].

11.3.1 Hodgkin's Lymphoma

A number of studies (Table 11.2) have investigated the safety of grafting cryopreserved human ovarian tissue from HL patients and suggest that ovarian tissue transplantation may be considered safe in this instance [6, 18–20].

One case report showed ovarian involvement in stage III HL [21], while another study [7] found the ovaries to be affected by HL in 4.3 % of autopsies.

Table 11.2 Experimental studies on the risk of transmitting malignant cells in case of lymphoma, divided into two groups, depending on pathology (HL or NHL)

		n =	Histology	IHC	Xenografting	Autografting (patients)
HL	Meirow et al. [18]	7	Negative	–	–	–
	Kim et al. [19]	13	Negative	–	16 weeks (no relapse)	–
	Seshadri et al. [20]	26	Negative	Neg	–	–
	Meirow et al. [6]	33	Negative	Neg ($n = 1$)	–	1 (no relapse)
NHL	Meirow et al. [6]	14	Negative			2 (no relapse)
	Kim et al. [19]	5	Negative	–	16 weeks (no relapse)	

All studies used histology, and some were completed by the addition of either immunohistochemistry or xenografting experiments. One study reported autografting results
IHC immunohistochemistry

In a series reporting 15 autotransplantations of ovarian tissue in HL patients, and none of them experienced disease recurrence post-grafting [22]. The maximum follow-up after autotransplantation in HL patients is now more than 11 years [23].

11.3.2 Non-Hodgkin's Lymphoma (Table 11.2)

Six autotransplantations of frozen-thawed ovarian tissue from NHL patients have been reported, with no signs of disease recurrence [22, 25–30].

Although Kyono et al. [7] reported a 9.8 % incidence of ovarian involvement in NHL, histology did not reveal the presence of any malignant cells in ovarian cortex in a number of studies [6, 19, 31]. Kim et al. [19] did not evidence any metastasis after xenografting tissue to SCID mice for 16 weeks ($n = 13$ patients with HL, $n = 5$ with NHL).

However, malignant cells were detected by histological evaluation in 3 out of 32 patients (6 %) with NHL (Fig. 11.1). NHL cells were identified by immunohistochemistry in the medulla (1/32) and cortex (1/32) [4] (Fig. 11.1). While the risk is low, it nevertheless exists and thus warrants further investigation [1].

11.4 Breast Cancer

The incidence of ovarian metastasis in breast cancer patients can vary between 13.2 % and 37.8 % [7, 32], but is more commonly observed in case of advanced-stage disease. Sanchez et al. [34] and Rosendhal et al. [35] analyzed frozen-thawed ovarian cortical biopsies from breast cancer patients. Neither study revealed any

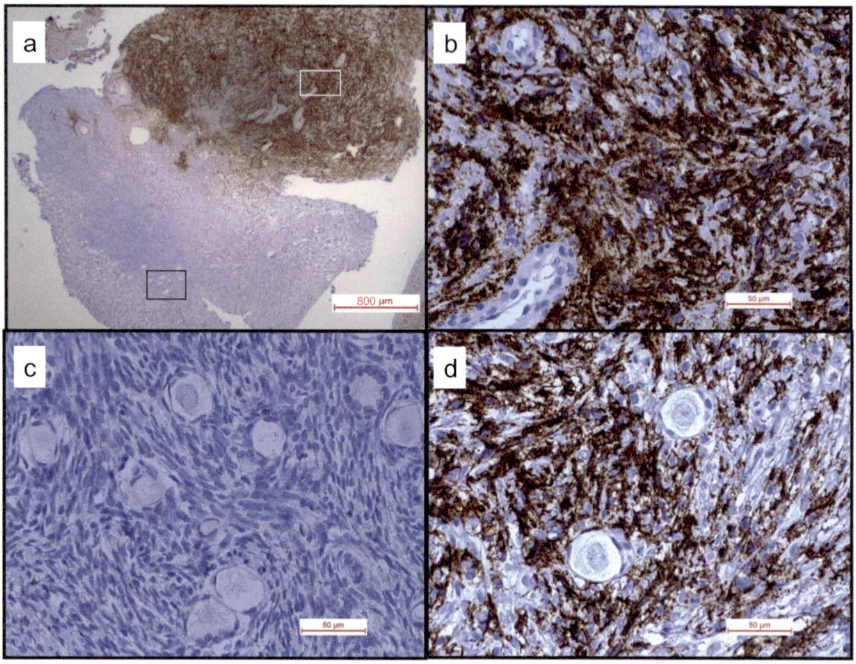

Fig. 11.1 Ovarian fragments from a non-Hodgkin's lymphoma patient. (**a**) Immunohistochemistry anti-CD20 (against NHL cells) is negative in the cortex (*blue*) and positive in the medulla (*brown* staining). The magnification of the *white rectangle* is represented in (**b**), and the magnification of the *black rectangle* is represented in (**c**). (**b**) Cells with an enlarged nucleus and patchy chromatin are disseminated in the tissue and stain strongly for anti-CD20. (**c**) Piece of cancer cell-free cortex. Follicles present in the cortex appear healthy. (**d**) Another fragment of the same patient shows massive invasion by NHL cells in the cortex

evidence of malignant cell infiltration of the cryopreserved ovarian tissue by histology or immunohistochemistry.

A third study by our group reported a series of 13 cases of advanced-stage breast cancer [36]. MGB2 gene expression was detected in five cases by RT-qPCR, but histology and immunohistochemistry failed to identify malignant cells in the ovarian tissue. The xenografted mice did not become ill [37].

A recent study by Demeester et al. [37] used the nGB1 gene as a molecular marker for detection of breast cancer cells in ovarian tissue. This shows that there is no standardization of detection methods as yet and the technique should be individualized according to each patient's primary disease. In conclusion, although these studies are encouraging, they nevertheless demonstrate that further procedures, such as PCR and long-term xenografting, are required to prove the safety of frozen-thawed ovarian tissue transplantation in women with advanced-stage breast cancer.

11.5 Cervical Carcinoma

It is well known that ovarian involvement is more frequent in adenocarcinoma than in squamous cell carcinoma. Ovarian metastasis has been reported in 0.7–2.5 % of patients with squamous cell carcinoma, but just 0–6.8 % of patients with adenocarcinoma of the cervix [38, 39].

Three patients with cervical cancer had their tissue heterotopically transplanted, one of whom suffered a pelvic relapse and died soon after transplantation [40]. No sign of relapse has so far been noted in either of the other two clinical cases published [29, 41, 42].

11.6 Endometrial Carcinoma

According to histological studies, the risk of ovarian metastasis with endometrial cancer ranges from 1.9 % (FIGO stage I tumors) [43] to 41.7 % (FIGO stage I–III tumors) [44].

11.7 Central Nervous System (CNS) Tumors

According to Sonmezer and Oktay [45], neuroblastoma is also classified as high risk for ovarian involvement, like leukemia.

Donnez et al. [46] performed reimplantation of frozen-thawed ovarian tissue in a patient cured of a metastatic neuroectodermal tumor of the orbit, who had her tissue cryopreserved prior to bone marrow transplantation. Histological evaluation of an ovarian sample before transplantation did not reveal ovarian metastasis, and the patient has now delivered her third child. She is now, however, relapsing locally (brain).

11.8 Sarcoma

The Danish team performed transplantation of cryopreserved ovarian tissue in a patient treated for Ewing's sarcoma [29, 47], who subsequently delivered a healthy baby twice.

Puberty was also induced in a young girl treated for Ewing's sarcoma by grafting her frozen-thawed ovarian tissue. Unfortunately, the patient relapsed and died. Andersen et al. [48] analyzed all the remaining fragments and failed to find any malignant cells by PCR.

Abir et al. [49] analyzed ovarian samples from eight patients with Ewing's sarcoma by histology, immunohistochemistry, and RT-qPCR. There was no evidence of the disease in ovaries from pathological studies ($n = 7$), but in one patient out of five, RT-qPCR proved positive for the Ewing's sarcoma translocation.

Poirot et al. [50] found no sign of ovarian metastasis in their histological studies of ovarian tissue from patients with Ewing's sarcoma, medulloblastoma, or neuroblastoma.

Histological analyses of ovarian tissue aiming to identify malignant cells in tissue from patients with bone sarcoma, osteosarcoma, and rhabdomyosarcoma are reassuring [31, 49], but it should be pointed out that some patients in these studies had already received chemotherapy before their ovarian tissue was frozen. Rosendahl et al. [51] xenotransplanted ovarian tissue from five patients with sarcoma, and no tumor invasion was detected.

11.9 Conclusion

Since the first published live birth, cryopreservation of ovarian tissue followed by orthotopic reimplantation has become the option of choice to restore fertility in women requiring immediate chemotherapy and in prepubertal patients [23]. This review evaluates the presence of malignant cells in ovarian tissue that could lead to recurrence of the primary disease after reimplantation. Sonmezer and Oktay [45] classified malignant diseases into three categories, representing low, intermediate, or high risk of ovarian involvement, which we slightly modified according to the recent literature, recategorizing Ewing's sarcoma and NHL from low to moderate risk (Table 11.3).

Among the different pathologies investigated, the highest risk of reimplanting malignant cells was found in case of leukemia. However, taking into account the findings of both Dolmans et al. [8, 12] and Greve et al. [11], the risk is likely to be very low if the ovarian cryopreservation procedure is carried out in women in complete remission. We strongly suggest that ovarian autotransplantation be discouraged when there is any risk of reimplanting malignant cells, especially in leukemia patients. In other pathologies, the risk is low, but it is vital to discuss it with patients before reimplantation, according to the classification presented in Table 11.3.

Table 11.3 Risk of ovarian metastasis according to cancer type

High risk	Moderate risk	Low risk
Leukemia	Breast cancer	Breast cancer
	Stage IV	*Stage I–II*
	Infiltrating lobular subtype	*Infiltrating ductal subtype*
Neuroblastoma	Colon cancer	Squamous cell carcinoma of the cervix
Burkitt lymphoma	Adenocarcinoma of the cervix	Hodgkin's lymphoma
	Non-Hodgkin's lymphoma	Osteogenic carcinoma
	Ewing's sarcoma	Non-genital rhabdomyosarcoma
		Wilm's tumor

Adapted from Sonmezer and Oktay [45], and modified by Dolmans according to the recent literature: Ewing's sarcoma and NHL recategorized from low to moderate risk

Acknowledgments The authors thank Mira Hryniuk, B.A., for reviewing the English language of the manuscript.

References

1. Donnez J, Dolmans MM (2013) Fertility preservation in women. Nat Rev Endocrinol 9:735–749
2. Donnez J, Dolmans MM (2014) Transplantation of ovarian tissue. Best Pract Res Clin Obstet Gynaecol 28:1188–1197
3. Donnez J, Dolmans MM (2015) Ovarian tissue freezing: current status. Curr Opin Obstet Gynecol 27:222–230
4. Dolmans MM, Luyckx V, Donnez J, Andersen CY, Greve T (2013) Risk of transferring malignant cells with transplanted frozen-thawed ovarian tissue. Fertil Steril 99:1514–1522
5. Dolmans MM, Jadoul P, Gilliaux S, Amorim AC, Luyckx V, Squifflet J, Donnez J, Van Langendonckt A (2013) A review of 15 years of ovarian tissue bank activities. J Assist Reprod Genet 30:305–314
6. Meirow D, Hardan I, Dor J, Fridman E, Elizur S, Ra'anani H, Slyusarevsky E, Amariglio N, Schiff E, Rechavi G, Nagler A, Yehuda B (2008) Searching for evidence of disease and malignant cell contamination in ovarian tissue stored from hematologic cancer patients. Hum Reprod 23:1007–1013
7. Kyono K, Doshida M, Toya M, Sato Y, Akahira J, Sasano H (2010) Potential indications for ovarian autotransplantation based on the analysis of 5571 autopsy finding of females under the age of 40 in Japan. Fertil Steril 93:2429–2430
8. Dolmans MM, Marinescu C, Saussoy P, Van LA, Amorim C, Donnez J (2010) Reimplantation of cryopreserved ovarian tissue from patients with acute lymphoblastic leukemia is potentially unsafe. Blood 116:2908–2914
9. Rosendahl M, Andersen MT, Ralfkiaer E, Kjeldsen L, Andersen MK, Andersen CY (2010) Evidence of residual disease in cryopreserved ovarian cortex from female patients with leukemia. Fertil Steril 94:2186–2190
10. Rosendahl M, Greve T, Andersen CY (2013) The safety of transplanting cryopreserved ovarian tissue in cancer patients: a review of the literature. J Assist Reprod Genet 30:11–24
11. Greve T, Clasen-Linde E, Andersen MT, Andersen MK, Rosendahl M, Ralfkiaer E, Yding Andersen C (2012) No signs of viable malignant cells in frozen-thawed ovarian cortex intended for fertility preservation from patients with leukaemia. Blood 120:4311–4316
12. Dolmans MM (2012) Safety of ovarian autotransplantation. Blood 120:4275–4276
13. Jahnukainen K, Tinkanen H, Wikström A, Dunkel L, Saarinen-Pihkala UM, Mäkinen S, Asadi Azarbaijani B, Oskam IC, Vettenranta K, Laine T, Kairisto V, Juvonen V (2012) Bone marrow remission status predicts leukemia contamination in ovarian biopsies collected for fertility preservation. Leukemia 27:1183–1185
14. Andolina JR, Neudorf SM, Corey SJ (2012) How I treat childhood CML. Blood 119:1821–1830
15. Goldman JM (2007) How I treat chronic myeloid leukemia in the imatinib era. Blood 110:2828–2837
16. Pye SM, Cortes J, Ault P, Hatfield A, Kantarjian H, Pilot R, Rosti G, Apperley JF (2008) The effects of imatinib on pregnancy outcome. Blood 15(111):5505–5508
17. Donnez J, Dolmans MM (2011) Preservation of fertility in females with haematological malignancy. Br J Haematol 154:175–184
18. Meirow D, Ben Yehuda D, Prus D et al (1998) Ovarian tissue banking in patients with Hodgkin's disease: is it safe? Fertil Steril 69:996–998

19. Kim SS, Radford J, Harris M et al (2001) Ovarian tissue harvested from lymphoma patients to preserve fertility may be safe for autotransplantation. Hum Reprod 16:2056–2060
20. Seshadri T, Gook D, Lade S et al (2006) Lack of evidence of disease contamination in ovarian tissue harvested for cryopreservation from patients with Hodgkin lymphoma and analysis of factors predictive of oocyte yield. Br J Cancer 94:1007–1010
21. Bittinger SE, Nazaretian SP, Good DA, Parmar C, Harrup RA, Stern CJ (2011) Detection of Hodgkin lymphoma within ovarian tissue. Fertil Steril 95:803.e3–6
22. Donnez J, Silber S, Andersen CY, Demeestere I, Piver P, Meirow D, Pellicer A, Dolmans MM (2011) Children born after autotransplantation of cryopreserved ovarian tissue. A review of 13 live births. Ann Med 43:437–450
23. Donnez J, Dolmans MM, Demylle D, Jadoul P, Pirard C, Squifflet J, Martinez-Madrid B, van Langendonckt A (2004) Livebirth after orthotopic transplantation of cryopreserved ovarian tissue. Lancet 364:1405–1410
24. Akar ME, Carrillo AJ, Jennell JL, Yalcinkaya TM (2011) Robotic assisted laparoscopic ovarian tissue transplantation. Fertil Steril 95:1120–1128
25. Meirow D, Levron J, Eldar-Geva T, Hardan I, Fridman E, Zalel Y et al (2005) Pregnancy after transplantation of cryopreserved ovarian tissue in a patient with ovarian failure after chemotherapy. N Engl J Med 353:318–321
26. Meirow D, Baum M, Yaron R, Levron J, Hardan I, Schiff E et al (2007) Ovarian tissue cryopreservation in hematologic malignancy: ten years' experience. Leuk Lymphoma 48:1569–1576
27. Stern CJ, Toledo MG, Hale LG, Gook DA, Edgar DH (2011) The first Australian experience of heterotopic grafting of cryopreserved ovarian tissue: evidence of establishment of normal ovarian function. Aust N Z J Obstet Gynaecol 51:268–275
28. Tryde Schmidt KL, Yding AC, Starup J, Loft A, Byskov AG, Nyboe AA (2004) Orthotopic autotransplantation of cryopreserved ovarian tissue to a woman cured of cancer—follicular growth, steroid production and oocyte retrieval. Reprod BioMed Online 8:448–453
29. Schmidt KT, Rosendahl M, Ernst E, Loft A, Andersen AN, Dueholm M et al (2011) Autotransplantation of cryopreserved ovarian tissue in 12 women with chemotherapy-induced premature ovarian failure: the Danish experience. Fertil Steril 95:695–701
30. Andersen CY, Rosendahl M, Byskov AG et al (2008) Two successful pregnancies following autotransplantation of frozen/thawed ovarian tissue. Hum Reprod 23:2266–2272
31. Azem F, Hasson J, Ben-Yosef D, Kossoy N, Cohen T, Almog B, Amit A, Lessing JB, Lifschitz-Mercer B (2010) Histologic evaluation of fresh human ovarian tissue before cryopreservation. Int J Gynecol Pathol 29:19–23
32. Perrotin F, Marret H, Bouquin R, Fischer-Perrotin N, Lansac J, Body G (2001) Incidence, diagnosis and prognosis of ovarian metastasis in breast cancer. Gynecol Obstet Fertil 29:308–315
33. Gagnon Y, Têtu B (1989) Ovarian metastases of breast carcinoma. A clinicopathologic study of 59 cases. Cancer 64:892–898
34. Sánchez-Serrano M, Novella-Maestre E, Roselló-Sastre E, Camarasa N, Teruel J, Pellicer A (2009) Malignant cells are not found in ovarian cortex from breast cancer patients undergoing ovarian cortex cryopreservation. Hum Reprod 24:2238–2243
35. Rosendahl M, Timmermans Wielenga V, Nedergaard L, Kristensen SG, Ernst E, Rasmussen PE, Anderson M, Schmidt KT, Andersen CY (2011) Cryopreservation of ovarian tissue for fertility preservation: no evidence of malignant cell contamination in ovarian tissue from patients with breast cancer. Fertil Steril 95:2158–2161
36. Luyckx V, Durant JF, Camboni A, Gilliaux S, Amorim CA, Van Langendonckt A, Irenge LM, Gala JL, Donnez J, Dolmans MM (2013) Is transplantation of cryopreserved ovarian tissue from patients with advanced-stage breast cancer safe? A pilot study. J Assist Reprod Genet 30:1289–1299
37. Bockstaele L, Boulenouar S, Van Den Steen G, Dechène J, Tsepelidis S, Craciun L, Noël JC, Demeestere I (2015) Evaluation of quantitative polymerase chain reaction markers for the

detection of breast cancer cells in ovarian tissue stored for fertility preservation. Fertil Steril 104(2):410–417

38. Morice P, Haie-Meder C, Pautier P, Lhomme C, Castaigne D (2001) Ovarian metastasis on transposed ovary in patients treated for squamous cell carcinoma of the uterine cervix: report of two cases and surgical implications. Gynecol Oncol 83:605–607
39. Nakanishi T, Wakai K, Ishikawa H, Nawa A, Suzuki Y, Nakamura S, Kuzuya K (2001) A comparison of ovarian metastasis between squamous cell carcinoma and adenocarcinoma of the uterine cervix. Gynecol Oncol 82:504–509
40. Kim SS (2012) Assessment of long term endocrine function after transplantation of frozen-thawed ovarian tissue to the heterotopic site: 10 year longitudinal follow-up study. J Assist Reprod Genet 29:489–493
41. Donnez J, Dolmans MM, Pellicer A, Diaz-Garcia C, Sanchez Serrano M, Schmidt KT, Ernst E, Luyckx V, Andersen CY (2013) Restoration of ovarian activity and pregnancy after transplantation of cryopreserved ovarian tissue: a review of 60 cases of reimplantation. Fertil Steril 99:1503–1513
42. Donnez J, Dolmans MM, Pellicer A, Diaz-Garcia C, Ernst E, Macklon KT, Andersen CY (2015) Fertility preservation for age-related fertility decline. Lancet 385:506–507
43. Pan Z, Wang X, Zhang X, Chen X, Xie X (2011) Retrospective analysis on coexisting ovarian cancer in 976 patients with clinical stage I endometrial carcinoma. J Obstet Gynaecol Res 37:352–358
44. Dundar E, Tel N, Ozalp SS, Isiksoy S, Kabukcuoglu S, Bal C (2002) The significance of local cellular immune response of women 50 years of age and younger with endometrial carcinoma. Eur J Gynaecol Oncol 23:243–246
45. Sonmezer M, Oktay K (2004) Fertility preservation in female patients. Hum Reprod Update 10:251–266
46. Donnez J, Squifflet J, Jadoul P, Demylle D, Cheron AC, Van Langendonckt A, Dolmans MM (2011) Pregnancy and live birth after autotransplantation of frozen-thawed ovarian tissue in a patient with metastatic disease undergoing chemotherapy and hematopoietic stem cell transplantation. Fertil Steril 95:1787
47. Ernst E, Bergholdt S, Jørgensen JS, Andersen CY (2010) The first woman to give birth to two children following transplantation of frozen/thawed ovarian tissue. Hum Reprod 25:1280–1281
48. Sørensen SD, Greve T, Wielenga VT, Wallace WH, Andersen CY (2014) Safety considerations for transplanting cryopreserved ovarian tissue to restore fertility in female patients who have recovered from Ewing's sarcoma. Future Oncol 10:277–283
49. Abir R, Feinmesser M, Yaniv I, Fisch B, Cohen IJ, Ben-Haroush A, Meirow D, Felz C, Avigad S (2010) Occasional involvement of the ovary in Ewing sarcoma. Hum Reprod 25:1708–1712
50. Poirot CJ, Martelli H, Genestie C, Golmard JL, Valteau-Couanet D, Helardot P, Pacquement H, Sauvat F, Tabone MD et al (2007) Feasibility of ovarian tissue cryopreservation for prepubertal females with cancer. Pediatr Blood Cancer 49:74–78
51. Rosendahl M, Schmidt KT, Ernst E, Rasmussen PE, Loft A, Byskov AG, Nyboe Andersen A, Andersen CY (2011) Cryopreservation of ovarian tissue for a decade in Denmark—an overview of the technique. Reprod Med Online 22:162–171

Chapter 12
Artificial Ovary

Christiani A. Amorim

Abstract Survival rates of many malignant diseases are steadily improving, but for patients of childbearing age, fertility restoration often becomes a vital concern after disease remission. In women, treatments such as chemo/radiotherapy can be very harmful to the ovaries, causing loss of both endocrine and reproductive functions. When gonadotoxic treatment cannot be delayed, ovarian tissue cryobanking is the only way of preserving fertility. However, this technique is not advisable for patients with certain types of cancer, since there is a risk of reintroducing malignant cells present in the cryopreserved tissue. For these patients, a safer alternative could be transplantation of isolated preantral follicles back to their natural environment. To encapsulate and protect isolated follicles, a transplantable artificial ovary needs to be created. The main goal of the artificial ovary is to mimic the natural organ, and for this, it should be composed of a matrix that encapsulates and protects not only the isolated follicles but also autologous ovarian cells and bioactive factors, which are necessary for follicle survival and development. The aim of this chapter is to describe this new technology, its indications, advantages, and the different approaches to create it.

Keywords Preantral follicles • Cancer patients • Fertility preservation • Ovary • Stromal cells

12.1 Introduction

12.1.1 Ovarian Tissue Cryopreservation and Transplantation to Restore Fertility in Cancer Patients

In recent years, advanced chemo/radiotherapeutic treatments have led to high survival rates in cancer patients, giving rise to new issues for cancer survivors. Indeed, one major concern is future fertility in these women, since they may face

C.A. Amorim (✉)
Pôle de Recherche en Gynécologie, Institut de Recherche Expérimentale et Clinique, Université Catholique de Louvain, Avenue Mounier 52, bte. B1.52.02, 1200 Brussels, Belgium
e-mail: christiani.amorim@uclouvain.be

N. Suzuki, J. Donnez (eds.), *Gonadal Tissue Cryopreservation in Fertility Preservation*, DOI 10.1007/978-4-431-55963-4_12

premature ovarian failure [1]. For this reason, different strategies have been proposed to preserve their fertility. When gonadotoxic treatment cannot be delayed, ovarian tissue cryobanking appears to be the most promising way of preserving a patient's fertility. Moreover, this is the sole means of safeguarding fertility in prepubertal girls. Autotransplantation is the only alternative able to restore ovarian function from cryopreserved ovarian tissue fragments in cancer survivors at present. So far, this technique has led to successful ovarian function restoration and more than 40 pregnancies in a number of centers around the world [2]. However, there is a real concern regarding the potential presence of malignant cells in the frozen-thawed fragments, which could cause a recurrence of the primary disease after grafting [3]. While various types of cancer never metastasize to the ovaries, leukemia is systemic in nature and poses a significant risk to the patient. On the other hand, breast cancer and some types of lymphoma are classed as moderate risk.

Worldwide leukemia incidence is around 352,254 cases per year, and it is the 12th most common cancer in Europe. The mean number of new cases per 100,000 women is 10.2, and 15 % of these patients are prepubertal girls and women of reproductive age (up to 34 years). Thanks to early diagnosis and improved treatments, only 5.5 % of these patients die [4, 5]. In our ovarian tissue cryobank at St Luc's University Hospital, around 11 % of stored ovarian biopsies come from patients with leukemia. Unfortunately, it is not possible to transplant tissue from these women after their health has been restored, due to the potential risk of transferring malignant cells.

12.1.2 In Vitro Culture of Preantral Follicles: An In Vitro Artificial Ovary

In vitro culture of ovarian fragments containing preantral follicles is an emerging assisted reproductive technology that could potentially be applied for fertility preservation in these patients. However, the process of follicle development from the primordial to the preovulatory stage, known as folliculogenesis, takes around 6 months in humans and is not yet fully understood. For this reason, research groups around the world have not been able to design the best conditions and media required for these follicles to grow in vitro during this long period of time. Even after decades of studies, this complex and challenging procedure has never been achieved using human follicles.

Besides being unable to confirm the feasibility of this technique, there is also the risk of very dangerous consequences with its application; indeed, such a long period of in vitro culture could interfere with epigenetic mechanisms and, in particular, genomic imprinting. It is important to bear in mind that aberrant imprinting is linked to cancer and also a number of human imprinting disorders, such as Beckwith-Wiedemann, Prader-Willi, and Angelman syndromes [6].

12.1.3 Transplantation of Isolated Preantral Follicles: A New Strategy

Since ex vivo folliculogenesis has never been accomplished in humans and may lead to serious consequences, a safer alternative could be transplantation of isolated preantral follicles back to their natural environment. As follicles are enclosed in a basement membrane that prevents direct contact between follicular cells and capillaries, white blood cells, and nerve processes [7], their isolation will ensure that no malignant cells are returned back to patients. To encapsulate and protect isolated follicles, a transplantable artificial ovary needs to be created.

12.2 Assembly of a Transplantable Artificial Ovary

The main goal of the transplantable artificial ovary is to mimic the natural organ in order to allow follicles to survive and grow. To this end, it is necessary to develop the physical aspects and biological properties of the original organ, which will be responsible for maintaining the original structure of follicles, ensuring proper communication between follicles and surrounding ovarian cells, preserving their interaction with the extracellular matrix (ECM), and supplying factors involved in follicular survival and development (Fig. 12.1).

In practice, the transplantable artificial ovary should be composed of a matrix that encapsulates and protects isolated preantral follicles. Such a matrix should also be able to embed autologous ovarian cells (from a new ovarian sample after cancer

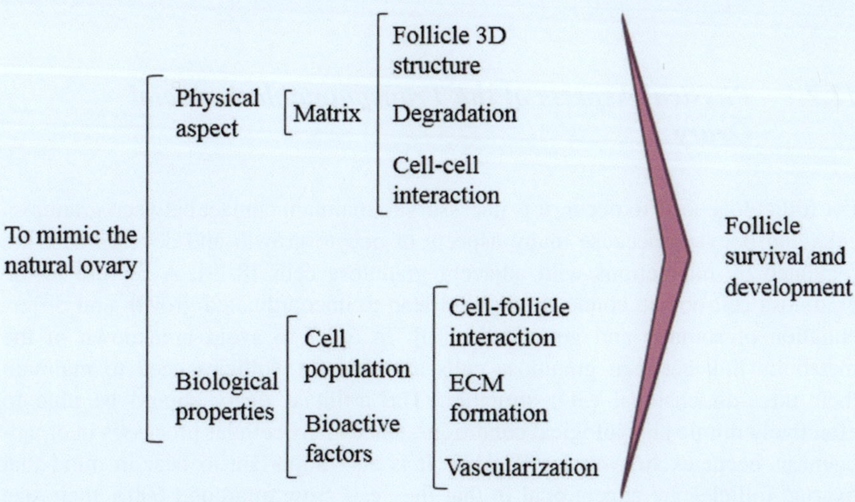

Fig. 12.1 Essential aspects of the transplantable artificial ovary required for survival and development of isolated preantral follicles

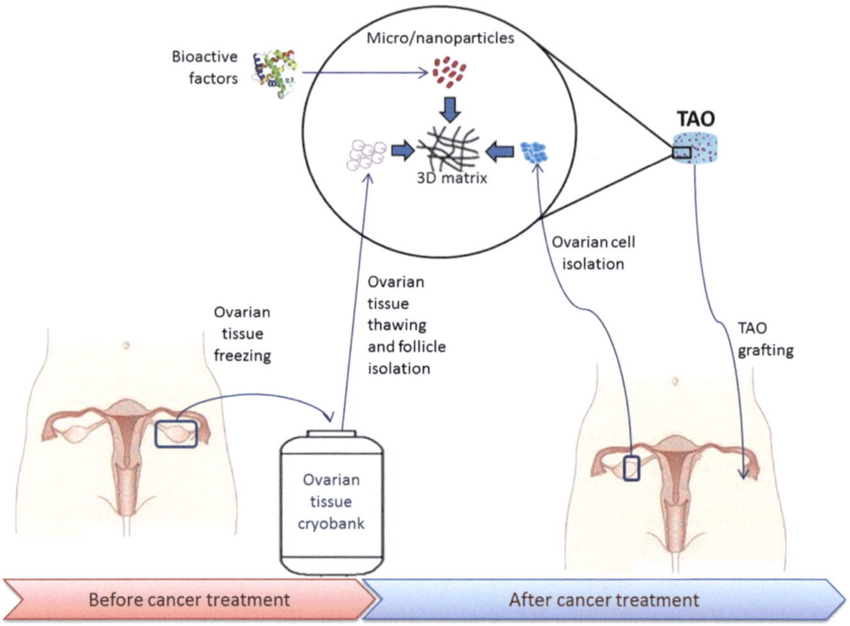

Fig. 12.2 Grafting of the transplantable artificial ovary containing isolated preantral follicles from frozen-thawed ovarian tissue, isolated ovarian cells from fresh ovarian biopsies, and micro-/nanoparticles with bioactive factors

treatment) and bioactive factors needed for follicle survival, development, and angiogenesis (Fig. 12.2).

12.2.1 Physical Aspects of the Transplantable Artificial Ovary

For folliculogenesis to occur, it is necessary to maintain contact between granulosa cells and oocytes, because many aspects of oocyte growth and development are regulated by interactions with adjacent granulosa cells [8, 9]. A rupture in the granulosa cell-oocyte connection would lead to uncoordinated growth and differentiation of somatic and germ cells [10]. In order to avoid breakdown of the metabolic link between granulosa cells and oocytes, follicles need to maintain their three-dimensional (3D) structure. The artificial ovary should be able to effectively mimic physiological conditions, since many cellular processes in organogenesis occur exclusively in 3D [11]. It is also important to bear in mind that ovarian follicles are exceptional in that they can grow to around 600× their size during folliculogenesis (for instance, the human follicle grows from 30 μm in its primordial stage to 18–24 mm when it is ready to ovulate). In addition, they recruit cells and vessels to support their development. Hence, the artificial ovary needs to degrade in order to allow exponential growth of follicles, formation of vessels, and proliferation of surrounding cells. Ideally, the artificial ovary should offer an appropriate initial environment for follicles that would be replaced by a new "ovary-like" structure after a few weeks of grafting.

With these features in mind, different materials have been tested to create the artificial ovary.

12.2.1.1 Plasma Clots

Pioneer studies on the grafting of isolated primordial follicles were conducted by Gosden [12], who first demonstrated the ability of dispersed ovarian cells (stromal cells and follicles) to reorganize into a functioning organ, allowing restoration of fertility after transplantation. In his study, Gosden [12] reported that mouse ovarian tissue can be enzymatically digested before being encapsulated in plasma clots and grafted to the ovarian bursa of sterile mice, where the ovarian digest is reorganized into morphologically normal ovaries. This experiment produced normal offspring, though litter size was small and graft longevity was relatively short. Carroll and Gosden [13] later proved that preantral follicles from frozen-thawed murine ovaries also have the ability to develop after isolation, encapsulation in plasma clots, and transplantation. The ovaries were capable of ovulating and host females delivered normal offspring.

Inspired by these successful results in mice [12, 13], Dolmans et al. [14, 15] xenografted enzymatically isolated human preantral follicles encapsulated in autologous plasma clots. After short-term xenografting, these follicles were able to survive and grow up to the secondary stage, and 5 months after xenografting, antral follicles could also be found. The most intriguing observation was the presence of stroma-like cells of human origin in isolated follicle grafts.

Despite these promising results, plasma clots remain difficult to handle, leading to follicle loss, and their unknown composition can yield variable outcomes.

12.2.1.2 Alginate

Alginate hydrogel has some attractive characteristics for artificial ovary application, including biodegradability, easy encapsulation of cells, and biocompatibility. Biodegradation of alginate hydrogels is normally slow, but certain processes can increase this rate, such as use of alginate lyase [16], an enzyme that hydrolyses alginate by cutting glycosidic links between monomers. This latter procedure has the advantage of being quantifiable and reproducible, since its concentration can be adjusted within the scaffold. Moreover, this enzyme can be encapsulated in poly (lactic-co-glycolic acid) (PLGA) microspheres, so alginate degradation can occur in a controlled manner [16]. Alginate also allows easy cell encapsulation. Droplets of alginate containing isolated cells can be extruded into millimolar concentrations of bivalent cations, such as calcium or barium, in order to form hydrogel beads [17]. This is particularly useful in the context of our application.

An alginate matrix that mimics the biophysical in vivo environment forms a rigid structure around cells, but allows their expansion due to proliferation. Indeed, such a matrix has been shown to preserve 3D follicle structure and enable growth of isolated preantral follicles after in vitro culture [18].

The first experiments using alginate to transplant isolated preantral follicles were performed by Vanacker et al. [16]. In their first study, they isolated ovarian cells and, after encapsulation in an alginate-matrigel matrix, carried out short-term autografting to mice. After this period of transplantation, they observed survival and proliferation of ovarian cells and formation of capillaries inside the remaining alginate-matrigel matrix. However, since matrigel cannot be used in a clinical setting, Vanacker et al. [19] replaced their alginate-matrigel matrix with a good manufacturing practice (GMP)-produced alginate (NovaMatrix 1 % SLM). They repeated the same experimental design, but also added isolated murine preantral follicles and grafted the matrix inside a peritoneal pocket (Fig. 12.3). After 1 week of autografting, 20 % of grafted follicles were found at more advanced stages of development (Fig. 12.4), and the alginate matrix was invaded by proliferating cells. However, it was not possible to control the degradation rate in this matrix, and as a result, vascularization inside the matrix was limited to its periphery.

12.2.1.3 Fibrin

Fibrin hydrogels are constituted from commercially purified allogeneic fibrinogen and purified thrombin [20]. They have been widely used in the last decade for a variety of tissue engineering applications in adipose [21], cardiovascular [22, 23], ocular [24, 25], muscle [26, 27], liver [28, 29], skin [30, 31], cartilage [32, 33], and bone [34, 35] tissues. Moreover, fibrin hydrogels are able to promote angiogenesis [36, 37].

However, varying concentrations of fibrinogen and thrombin can influence the morphology and rigidity of the fibrin network, and thereby cell survival and proliferation [38, 39]. Based on this observation, Luyckx et al. [40] decided to develop a fibrin matrix that would allow survival and proliferation of isolated human ovarian cells by determining the optimal combination of fibrinogen and thrombin. Taking into account matrix handling and cell survival, density, and proliferation, Luyckx et al. [40] found that two fibrin compositions with low concentrations of fibrinogen and thrombin showed the greatest distribution of cells before in vitro culture, reproducible degradation of the fibrin network, and adequate support for isolated human ovarian stromal cells, with a high proportion of proliferating cells.

Following this first step to build a 3D biodegradable fibrin-based artificial ovary, Luyckx et al. [41] compared these two fibrin formulations by autografting isolated murine preantral follicles. After 1 week, the follicle recovery rate was around 31 %. With both fibrin formulations, all follicles were found to be alive or minimally

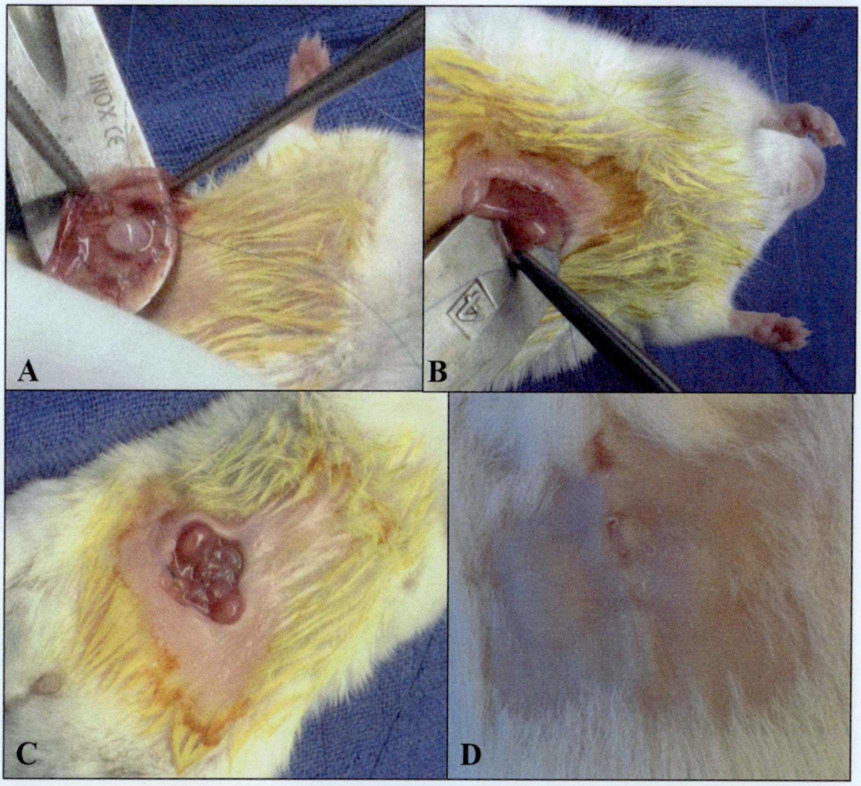

Fig. 12.3 Grafting of the matrix containing isolated preantral follicles and isolated ovarian cells. The matrix is first placed in the middle of a circle stitched with nonabsorbable 6/0 Prolene (**a**) thread. Then, with the aid of forceps, the peritoneum is folded over itself, and the ends of the thread are pulled in order to close the pocket and capture the matrix inside (**b**). Two pockets (*arrows*) can be made in each mouse (**c**). View of the grafted matrices (*arrows*) after 1 week of grafting (**d**)

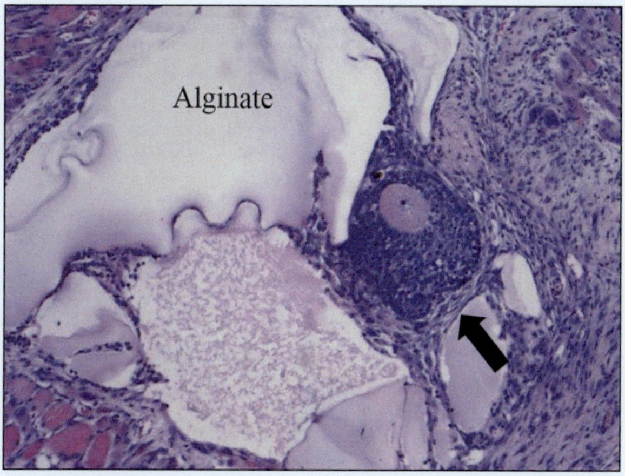

Fig. 12.4 Isolated murine secondary follicle recovered after 1 week of grafting inside an alginate matrix

damaged and at the growing stage (primary, secondary, and antral follicles). Isolated ovarian cells also survived and proliferated after grafting. Unlike with the alginate matrix [19], vessels were found not only at the periphery of the matrix, but also inside the fibrin clots.

Using higher concentrations of fibrinogen and thrombin, Smith et al. [42] grafted isolated murine preantral follicles inside the ovarian bursa for 3 weeks. They reported a significant increase in the population of secondary follicles and the appearance of antral follicles by the end of the grafting period. The presence of corpora lutea and decrease in follicle-stimulating hormone (FSH) levels showed that the grafts were able to restore hormone cyclicity.

Nevertheless, it is important to bear in mind that fibrin hydrogel has three major disadvantages as a potential scaffold: (1) shrinkage of the gel that occurs during formation of flat sheets, (2) a low degree of mechanical stiffness, and (3) rapid degradation before proper formation of tissue-engineered structures [43].

12.2.1.4 Decellularized Ovarian ECM

In recent years, decellularized tissues/organs have attracted much attention in the fields of tissue engineering and regenerative medicine. This concept involves decellularization of allogeneic or xenogeneic homologous tissue or organ followed by recellularization of the resultant 3D scaffold with autologous cells [44]. Three-dimensional decellularized tissue consists exclusively of the component molecules of ECM, ideally preserved in their native ultrastructural architecture. Decellularization techniques have led to the development of scaffolds for multiple organs, including the heart, liver, lungs, and kidneys [45].

Laronda et al. [46] constructed scaffolds from decellularized bovine and human ovarian tissue to graft primary murine ovarian cells. These recellularized matrices were able to initiate puberty in host ovariectomized mice.

Another application of decellularized tissue is its use in the manufacture of hydrogels. Decellularized ECM-based hydrogels can promote de novo formation of functional tissue [47], as they retain their biological activity and encourage tissue regeneration [48]. Indeed, after removal of the cellular components, an array of ECM proteins present in native tissue remains in the acellular hydrogel [48]. Another advantage of these hydrogels is that cytokines stored in tissues or cells at the time of decellularization can also be preserved [49]. Such cytokines may promote tissue growth because they can be released into regenerating tissue as the hydrogel is remodeled [48]. In a preliminary study, Viswanath et al. [50] developed a decellularization method to produce a soluble form of ECM from bovine ovaries that could be induced to form a hydrogel. After decellularization and solubilization, they reported that 89 % of the hydrogel was composed of collagen. They also calculated the storage modulus and viscous modulus of decellularized ovarian ECM hydrogel and used it for in vitro culture of mouse primary follicles. After 10 days of culture, the follicles remained viable in the hydrogels (Fig. 12.5).

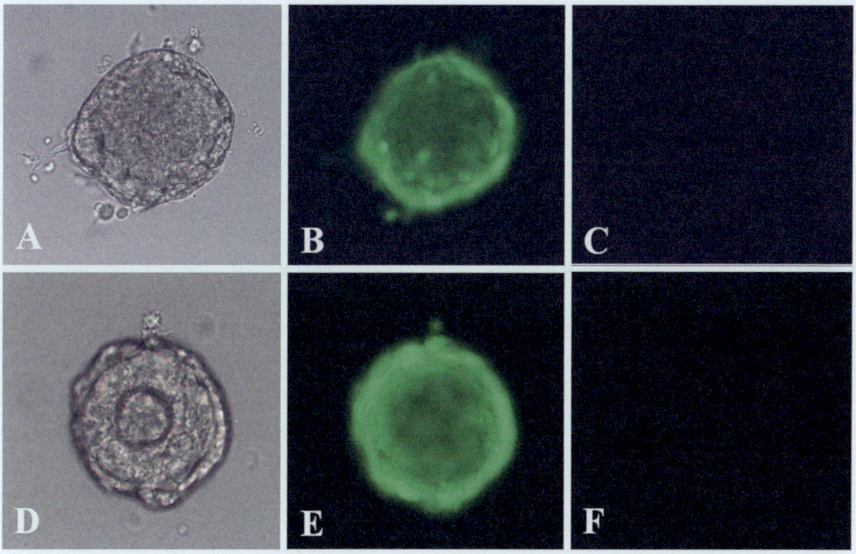

Fig. 12.5 Isolated preantral follicles before (**a–c**) and after (**d–f**) 7 days of in vitro culture. The *second* and *third columns* show follicle viability assessment by calcein AM and ethidium homodimer-I

12.2.2 Biological Properties of the Transplantable Artificial Ovary

12.2.2.1 Cell Population

Ovarian stromal cells are essential for early folliculogenesis. They provide structural support and show complex bidirectional paracrine signaling with follicles [51], and those adjacent to follicles are recruited to differentiate into theca cells, which play an essential role in follicular development through secretion of androgens [52]. Integration of ovarian cells into the artificial ovary could thus serve to better simulate the ovarian microenvironment and potentially improve follicle growth and survival.

Ovarian (stromal and endothelial) cells for the artificial ovary could be isolated, like follicles, from ovarian cortex cryopreserved before chemotherapy. In this case, stromal cells would have to undergo malignant cell purging before they could be safely used. An alternative is to take a fresh ovarian biopsy (cortex and/or medulla) just before transplantation of the artificial ovary, once the patient is disease-free. These ovarian cells isolated from fresh ovarian tissue would then be combined with follicles obtained from cryopreserved cortex and would not require malignant cell purging.

Soares et al. [53] evaluated the best source of ovarian cells to be grafted inside the artificial ovary: cortex or medulla, cryopreserved or fresh. Their findings suggest that ovarian cells from fresh medullary tissue can be isolated in larger numbers, show higher viability, and are able to improve graft vascularization.

In another study on the grafting of isolated ovarian cells, Dath et al. [54] showed that the presence of stromal cells isolated from human ovarian tissue can increase matrix degradation and form an ovary-like structure after xenografting. However, we do not know whether such stromal cells would have the same ability to differentiate into theca cells as those surrounding follicles. A study performed with bovine cells indicates that this may be possible; Orisaka et al. [55] demonstrated that bovine cortical stromal cells can differentiate into theca cells under the influence of granulosa cells.

Another requirement for follicle survival and growth is vascularization. Vascular development is therefore crucial during the first month after transplantation, and for this, it is necessary to promote angiogenesis in the hypoxic environment for follicle engraftment. In this context, endothelial cells appear to play a vital role, aiding survival of several types of cells by improving the quality of revascularization after transplantation [56]. Dath et al. [54] demonstrated the importance of co-transplanting ovarian endothelial cells and stromal cells to ensure formation of a well vascularized and structured ovary-like stroma after grafting.

12.2.2.2 Bioactive Factors

Folliculogenesis in humans is a long and poorly understood process. For instance, it is not known which factors play a role in the activation of primordial follicles and initial growth of primary follicles. For creation of the artificial ovary, it is essential to determine which factors are implicated in these early stages of folliculogenesis, so that it can be controlled from the very first moments after artificial ovary transplantation to ensure follicle survival and correct development. There are currently no studies on gene expression dynamics during ovarian folliculogenesis in humans.

Another important concern is how growth factors could be incorporated into the artificial ovary in a way that would safeguard their activity and avoid denaturation and degradation over a shorter period of time. Several studies on the influence of different growth factors on in vitro development of human follicles have shown contradictory results [57]. This is probably due to addition of the factors directly to the culture media, which could have altered their effect on follicles. Moreover, since follicles require different factors at different periods of their development, release of these factors should take place at different time points. For this, they need to be encapsulated in degradable nano-/microparticles. Their release may be modulated by the quantity encapsulated in microspheres, by the number of microspheres incorporated in the artificial ovary, or by the composition of the microspheres. Moreover, microspheres containing different factors implicated in follicle recruitment and development can be tested in order to understand the intricate mechanisms involved in folliculogenesis. Another advantage of encapsulation is that it can protect these factors from denaturation that could occur if they were directly adsorbed onto the artificial ovary, which would result in their complete degradation in a very short period of time.

In this way, inhibitory factors, such as anti-Müllerian hormone (AMH), could be encapsulated in microspheres, and their slow release would ensure recruitment of just a few primordial follicles at a time, preventing activation of the remaining follicular pool. This could considerably increase graft life span. On the other hand, growth factors like vascular endothelial growth factor (VEGF) could also be incorporated, with the aim of increasing vessel formation around and inside the graft. This would favor transport of oxygen, nutrients, and degradation products in the scaffold, enhancing survival and development of the encapsulated follicles and stromal cells.

12.3 Other Important Aspects to Consider: Safety

A number of protocols have been developed to isolate human preantral follicles [58, 59] for further transplantation. A technique for isolation of human preantral follicles following GMP conditions was recently optimized by Vanacker et al. [60] with a view to clinical application.

However, even if isolation of preantral follicles from ovarian cortex in healthy women is now a well established protocol, caution must be exercised in women with cancer. Indeed, it cannot be excluded that some malignant cells could contaminate isolated follicle suspensions obtained from patients with leukemia. Based on this assumption, Soares et al. [61] reported a technique to effectively eliminate cancer cells from the follicle suspension without altering follicle viability. They found that in case of contamination of ovarian tissue by malignant cells, there is a real risk of picking up cancer cells along with isolated follicles during follicle retrieval. However, this risk is dramatically reduced when a simple mechanical procedure is added: manual pipetting of follicles, with transfer to fresh medium droplets, in order to remove unwanted contaminating cells. Repeating this procedure three times led to successful elimination of leukemic cells from the follicle suspension [61].

Because Soares et al. [61] detected leukemic cell contamination of the follicle suspension after pickup, they conducted another study to investigate the leukemia-inducing potential of a few leukemic cells grafted inside an artificial ovary environment using an immunodeficient mouse xenografting model [62]. Leukemic cells were embedded in a fibrin matrix along with ovarian cells in order to study leukemic cell survival and proliferation in conditions resembling the artificial ovary environment as closely as possible. After xenotransplantation, the authors reported that mice grafts with a fibrin matrix containing 10 or 100 leukemic cells did not show any signs of leukemia after 20 weeks [62], indicating that transplantation of such small numbers of leukemic cells appears to be insufficient to induce the disease. However, for clinical application, follicle suspensions must be completely purged of leukemic cells prior to grafting, as even the slightest risk must be avoided.

12.4 Advantages of the Transplantable Artificial Ovary

Although the main objective is to be able to provide an alternative means of restoring fertility in patients who cannot undergo ovarian tissue transplantation, the assembly and grafting of an artificial ovary would offer additional advantages compared to transplantation of ovarian tissue [63].

12.4.1 Improvement of Follicular Survival by Decreasing the Ischemic Period

After removal, freezing, thawing, and transplantation, ovarian tissue is subjected to hypoxia in the first few days post-grafting, and this deprivation of oxygen and nutrients, as well as accumulation of metabolic waste, may result in cellular damage. Indeed, it has been estimated that a significant percentage (50–95 %) of primordial follicles may be lost due to ischemia [64–66], which would directly affect the life span of the graft. Therefore, the success of primordial follicle transplantation depends on the growth of new blood vessels in order to restore adequate perfusion. This may be improved by the use of a scaffold with a porous structure, loaded with factors known to promote angiogenesis. An interconnected pore network in a scaffold has been shown to enhance vascularization in prostheses implanted in the abdominal aorta of rats [67], while appropriate pore size and distribution would facilitate diffusion of metabolites, oxygen and growth factors [68], which would have a positive effect on follicle survival and development. Angiogenic factors could also be added to the scaffold, either chemically immobilized or physically entrapped [68]. Shi et al. [69] conducted studies to develop an artificial dermis and showed that when angiogenin, a polypeptide involved in angiogenesis, was added to a porous collagen-chitosan scaffold subcutaneously grafted to rabbits, vascularization increased. Basic fibroblast growth factor (b-FGF) was also found to have a positive impact on vascularization in different studies. Peters et al. [70] observed almost fourfold faster vascularization when PLGA microspheres were loaded with b-FGF. These authors reported that released b-FGF induced the formation of large and mature blood vessels in scaffolds implanted in the mesenteric membrane of rats. Tanihara et al. [71] also described induction of angiogenesis by b-FGF in heparin/alginate scaffolds grafted to the dorsal area of rats. VEGF and platelet-derived growth factor (PDGF) were found to increase vessel density, size, and maturity when added to scaffolds grafted to mice [72]. According to Bergmann and West [68], these factors could well influence the differentiation of mesenchymal stem cells from the bloodstream into endothelial cells and encourage microvascularization.

12.4.2 Control of Follicular Development

It has also been suggested that premature recruitment of primordial follicles may occur after grafting of ovarian tissue, possibly caused by a deficiency in inhibitory mechanisms implicated in the quiescence of primordial follicles in intact ovaries [73]. This is indeed very likely, since tissue collected for cryopreservation and transplantation comes from the ovarian cortex, where the vast majority of the follicular population is made up of primordial and primary follicles, and there is a lack of larger follicles responsible for production of inhibitory factors like AMH and activin A. Using a scaffold, follicular activation and development may be modulated through supplementation of inhibitory and growth factors implicated in the different stages of folliculogenesis. These factors could, for example, be encapsulated in materials with different degradation rates, according to requirements after transplantation.

12.4.3 Improvement of Follicular Growth Using Fresh Ovarian Cells

Apart from the necessary interaction between granulosa cells and oocytes, follicles require neighboring stromal cells to support their growth. These cells are recruited to differentiate into theca cells, which play an essential role in follicular development through secretion of androgens, as well as improving perifollicular vascularity. Although freezing of ovarian tissue does not negatively affect the morphology or ultrastructural characteristics of primordial follicles [74], it is harmful to the surrounding tissue, causing damage to the ECM and stromal cell necrosis [75] and resulting in large areas of fibrosis [76]. The poor cellularity of tissue after freezing may affect the development of follicles and could be implicated in the lack of a structured theca layer around secondary follicles and asynchrony between oocyte and follicular cell growth [77]. Therefore, in order to improve follicular development in the scaffold, a fragment of ovarian tissue could be removed before the scaffold is grafted, with the aim of isolating fresh stromal cells. These cells would then be combined with isolated follicles from frozen tissue and seeded in the scaffold.

12.4.4 Control of the Number and Quality of Follicles to Be Grafted

Due to the random distribution of primordial follicles in ovarian cortex, it is not possible to determine the number, or even the presence, of follicles in ovarian tissue to be transplanted to a patient [18], which could affect the life span of the graft. Grafting isolated follicles would allow not only the introduction of a high and known number of follicles into the host [78] but also the assessment of follicular quality before grafting [79].

12.5 Conclusions

The transplantable artificial ovary may potentially have a huge impact on the quality of life of patients, as it will enable them to fulfill their dream of becoming mothers. Because it will allow them to conceive naturally, the artificial ovary will benefit the healthcare system, cutting expenses involved in oocyte donation, in vitro fertilization, and surrogacy programs. There is clearly a demand for this technology, as the artificial ovary will herald the dawn of a brand new therapy, not only for patients at risk of ovarian metastasis but also for other cancer sufferers, in whom it can replace transplantation of ovarian tissue.

This innovative medical technology could also be applied to patients with certain genetic or metabolic diseases that lead to premature ovarian failure and women opting to defer motherhood for social reasons or those looking to delay menopause for health reasons. Consequently, it will involve a growing number of subjects, given the increasing development and implementation of ovarian tissue cryobanks in centers of reproductive medicine around the world.

References

1. Donnez J, Martinez-Madrid B, Jadoul P et al (2006) Ovarian tissue cryopreservation and transplantation: a review. Hum Reprod Update 12:519–535
2. Donnez J, Dolmans MM (2013) Fertility preservation in women. Nat Rev Endocrinol 9:735–749. doi:10.1038/nrendo.2013.205
3. Meirow D, Hardan I, Dor J et al (2008) Searching for evidence of disease and malignant cell contamination in ovarian tissue stored from hematologic cancer patients. Hum Reprod 23:1007–1013. doi:10.1093/humrep/den055
4. SEER Stat Fact Sheets: leukemia. In: USA National Cancer Institute at the National Institutes of Health. http://seer.cancer.gov/statfacts/html/leuks.html. Accessed 10 May 2015
5. Leukaemia (all subtypes combined) statistics. In: Cancer Research UK. http://www.cancerresearchuk.org/health-professional/cancer-statistics/statistics-by-cancer-type/leukaemia. Accessed 10 May 2015

6. Lim DH, Maher ER (2010) Genomic imprinting syndromes and cancer. Adv Genet 70:145–175. doi:10.1016/B978-0-12-380866-0.60006-X
7. Rodgers RJ, Irving-Rodgers HF, Russell DL (2003) Extracellular matrix of the developing ovarian follicle. Reproduction 126:415–424
8. Murray AA, Gosden RG, Allison V et al (1998) Effect of androgens on the development of mouse follicles growing in vitro. J Reprod Fertil 113:27–33
9. Reynaud K, Cortvrindt R, Smitz J et al (2000) Effects of kit ligand and anti-kit antibody on growth of cultured mouse preantral follicles. Mol Reprod Dev 56:483–494
10. Picton HM, Gosden RG (2000) Mol Cell Endocrinol 166:27–35
11. Xu M, Kreeger PK, Shea LD et al (2006) Tissue-engineered follicles produce live, fertile offspring. Tissue Eng 12:2739–2746
12. Gosden RG (1990) Restitution of fertility in sterilized mice by transferring primordial ovarian follicles. Hum Reprod 5:499–504
13. Carroll J, Gosden RG (1993) Transplantation of frozen-thawed mouse primordial ovarian follicles. Hum Reprod 8:1163–1167
14. Dolmans MM, Martinez-Madrid B, Gadisseux E et al (2007) Short-term transplantation of isolated human ovarian follicles and cortical tissue into nude mice. Reproduction 134:253–262
15. Dolmans MM, Yuan WY, Camboni A et al (2008) Development of antral follicles after xenografting of isolated small human preantral follicles. Reprod Biomed Online 16:705–711
16. Vanacker J, Luyckx V, Dolmans MM et al (2012) Transplantation of an alginate-matrigel matrix containing isolated ovarian cells: first step in developing a biodegradable scaffold to transplant isolated preantral follicles and ovarian cells. Biomaterials 33:6079–6085. doi:10.1016/j.biomaterials.2012.05.015
17. Orive G, Carcaboso AM, Hernández RM et al (2005) Biocompatibility evaluation of different alginates and alginate-based microcapsules. Biomacromolecules 6:927–931
18. Amorim CA, Van Langendonckt A, David A et al (2009) Survival of human preantral follicles after cryopreservation of ovarian tissue, follicular isolation and in vitro culture in a calcium alginate matrix. Hum Reprod 24:92–99. doi:10.1093/humrep/den343
19. Vanacker J, Dolmans MM, Luyckx V et al (2014) First transplantation of isolated murine follicles in alginate. Regen Med 9:609–619. doi:10.2217/rme.14.33
20. Ahmed TA, Griffith M, Hincke M (2007) Characterization and inhibition of fibrin hydrogel-degrading enzymes during development of tissue engineering scaffolds. Tissue Eng 13:1469–1477
21. Cho SW, Kim I, Kim SH et al (2006) Enhancement of adipose tissue formation by implantation of adipogenic-differentiated preadipocytes. Biochem Biophys Res Commun 345:588–594
22. Birla RK, Borschel GH, Dennis RG et al (2005) Myocardial engineering in vivo: formation and characterization of contractile, vascularized three-dimensional cardiac tissue. Tissue Eng 11:803–813
23. Mol A, van Lieshout MI, Dam-de Veen CG et al (2005) Fibrin as a cell carrier in cardiovascular tissue engineering applications. Biomaterials 26:3113–3121
24. Alaminos M, Del Carmen Sanchez-Quevedo M, Munoz-Avila JI et al (2006) Construction of a complete rabbit cornea substitute using fibrin-agarose scaffold. Invest Ophthalmol Vis Sci 47:3311–3317
25. Suuronen EJ, Muzakare L, Doillon CJ et al (2006) Promotion of angiogenesis in tissue engineering: developing multicellular matrices with multiple capacities. Int J Artif Organs 29:1148–1157
26. Nieponice A, Maul TM, Cumer JM et al (2007) Mechanical stimulation induces morphological and phenotypic changes in bone marrow-derived progenitor cell within a three-dimensional fibrin matrix. J Biomed Mater Res A 81:523–530
27. Rowe SL, Lee S, Stegemann JP (2007) Influence of thrombin concentration on the mechanical and morphological properties of cell-seeded fibrin hydrogels. Acta Biomater 3:59–67
28. Bruns H, Kneser U, Holzhuter S et al (2005) Injectable liver: a novel approach using fibrin as a matrix for culture and intrahepatic transplantation of hepatocytes. Tissue Eng 11:1718–1726

29. Sun T, Chan ML, Quek CH et al (2004) Improving mechanical stability and density distribution of hepatocytes microcapsules by fibrin clot and gold nanoparticles. J Biotechnol 111:169–177
30. Balestrini JL, Billiar KL (2006) Equibiaxial cyclic stretch stimulates fibroblasts to rapidly remodel fibrin. J Biochem 39:2983–2990
31. Hojo M, Inokuchi S, Kidokoro M et al (2003) Induction of vascular endothelial growth factor by a fibrin as dermal substrate for cultured skin substitutes. Plast Reconstr Surg 111:1638–1645
32. Eyrich D, Brandle F, Appel B et al (2007) Long-term stable fibrin gels for cartilage engineering. Biomaterials 28:55–65
33. Mesa JM, Zaporojan V, Weinand C et al (2006) Tissue engineering cartilage with aged articular chondrocytes in vivo. Plast Reconstr Surg 118:41–49
34. Chung YI, Ahn KM, Jeo SH et al (2007) Enhanced bone regeneration with BMP-2 loaded functional nanoparticles-hydrogel complex. J Control Release 121:91–99
35. Weinand C, Pomerantseva I, Neville CM et al (2006) Hydrogel-b-TCP scaffolds and stem cells for tissue engineering bone. Bone 38:555–563
36. Liu JY, Swartz DD, Peng HF et al (2007) Functional tissue-engineered blood vessels from bone marrow progenitor cells. Cardiovasc Res 75:618–628
37. Dietrich F, Lelkes PI (2006) Fine-tuning of a three-dimensional microcarrier-based angiogenesis assay for the analysis of endothelial-mesenchymal cell co-cultures in fibrin and collagen gels. Angiogenesis 9:111–125
38. Ho W, Tawil B, Dunn JC et al (2006) The behavior of human mesenchymal stem cells in 3D fibrin clots: dependence on fibrinogen concentration and clot structure. Tissue Eng 12:1587–1595
39. Sese N, Cole M, Tawil B (2011) Proliferation of human keratinocytes and cocultured human keratinocytes and fibroblasts in three-dimensional fibrin constructs. Tissue Eng A 17:429–437. doi:10.1089/ten.TEA.2010.0113
40. Luyckx V, Dolmans MM, Vanacker J et al (2013) First step in developing a 3D biodegradable fibrin scaffold for an artificial ovary. J Ovarian Res 6:83. doi:10.1186/1757-2215-6-83
41. Luyckx V, Dolmans MM, Vanacker J et al (2014) A new step toward the artificial ovary: survival and proliferation of isolated murine follicles after autologous transplantation in a fibrin scaffold. Fertil Steril 101:1149–1156. doi:10.1016/j.fertnstert.2013.12.025
42. Smith RM, Shikanov A, Kniazeva E et al (2014) Fibrin-mediated delivery of an ovarian follicle pool in a mouse model of infertility. Tissue Eng A 20:3021–3030. doi:10.1089/ten.TEA.2013.0675
43. Ahmed TA, Dare EV, Hincke M (2008) Fibrin: a versatile scaffold for tissue engineering applications. Tissue Eng B Rev 14:199–215. doi:10.1089/ten.teb.2007.0435
44. Faulk DM, Johnson SA, Zhang L et al (2014) Role of the extracellular matrix in whole organ engineering. J Cell Physiol 229:984–989. doi:10.1002/jcp.24532
45. Arenas-Herrera JE, Ko IK, Atala A et al (2013) Decellularization for whole organ bioengineering. Biomed Mater 8:014106. doi:10.1088/1748-6041/8/1/014106
46. Laronda MM, Jakus AE, Whelan KA (2015) Initiation of puberty in mice following decellularized ovary transplant. Biomaterials 50:20–29. doi:10.1016/j.biomaterials.2015.01.051
47. Badylak SF, Brown BN, Gilbert TW et al (2011) Biologic scaffolds for constructive tissue remodeling. Biomaterials 32:316–319
48. Hoganson DM, Owens GE, O'Doherty E et al (2010) Preserved extracellular matrix components and retained biological activity in decellularized porcine mesothelium. Biomaterials 31:6934–6940. doi:10.1016/j.biomaterials.2010.05.026
49. Voytik-Harbin SL, Brightman AO, Kraine MR et al (1997) Identification of extractable growth factors from small intestinal submucosa. J Cell Biochem 67:478–491

50. Viswanath A, Germain L, Shakesheff K et al (2015) Hydrogen derived from decellularized bovine ovarian extracellular matrix; (Abstract 1492). Presented at the 4th TERMIS World Congress, 8 September 2015, Boston, MA, USA
51. Tagler DJ, Shea LD, Woodruff TK (2011) Contributions of ovarian cells to follicle culture. In: Donnez J, Kim SS (eds) Principles and practice of fertility preservation, 1st edn. Cambridge University Press, Cambridge, pp 409–420
52. Young JM, McNeilly AS (2010) Theca: the forgotten cell of the ovarian follicle. Reproduction 140:489–504. doi:10.1530/REP-10-0094
53. Soares M, Sahrari K, Chiti MC et al (2015) The best source of isolated stromal cells for the artificial ovary: medulla or cortex, cryopreserved or fresh? Hum Reprod 30(7):1589–1598
54. Dath C, Dethy A, Van Langendonckt A et al (2011) Endothelial cells are essential for ovarian stromal tissue restructuring after xenotransplantation of isolated ovarian stromal cells. Hum Reprod 26:1431–1439. doi:10.1093/humrep/der073
55. Orisaka M, Tajima K, Mizutani T et al (2006) Granulosa cells promote differentiation of cortical stromal cells into theca cells in the bovine ovary. Bio Reprod 75:734–740
56. Dudás J, Ramadori G, Knittel T (2000) Effect of heparin and liver heparan sulphate on interaction of HepG2-derived transcription factors and their cis-acting elements: altered potential of hepatocellular carcinoma heparan sulphate. Biochem J 1:245–251
57. Smitz J, Dolmans MM, Donnez J et al (2010) Current achievements and future research directions in ovarian tissue culture, in vitro follicle development and transplantation: implications for fertility preservation. Hum Reprod Update 16:395–414. doi:10.1093/humupd/dmp056
58. Dolmans MM, Michaux N, Camboni A et al (2006) Evaluation of Liberase, a purified enzyme blend, for the isolation of human primordial and primary ovarian follicles. Hum Reprod 21:413–420
59. Laronda MM, Duncan FE, Hornick JE et al (2014) Alginate encapsulation supports the growth and differentiation of human primordial follicles within ovarian cortical tissue. J Assist Reprod Genet 31:1013–1028
60. Vanacker J, Camboni A, Dath C et al (2011) Enzymatic isolation of human primordial and primary ovarian follicles with Liberase DH: protocol for application in a clinical setting. Fertil Steril 96:379–383.e3. doi:10.1016/j.fertnstert.2011.05.075
61. Soares M, Sahrari K, Amorim CA et al (2015) Evaluation of a human ovarian follicle isolation technique to obtain disease-free follicle suspensions before safely grafting to cancer patients. Fertil Steril 104(3):672–680.e2
62. Soares M, Saussoy P, Sahrari K et al (2015) Is transplantation of a few leukemic cells inside an artificial ovary able to induce leukemia in an experimental model? J Assist Reprod Genet 32:597–606. doi:10.1007/s10815-015-0438-x
63. Amorim CA (2011) Artificial ovary. In: Donnez J, Kim SS (eds) Principles and practice of fertility preservation, 1st edn. Cambridge University Press, Cambridge, pp 448–458
64. Newton H, Aubard Y, Rutherford et al (1996) Low temperature storage and grafting of human ovarian tissue. Hum Reprod 11:1487–1491
65. Aubard Y, Piver P, Cogni Y et al (1999) Orthotopic and heterotopic autografts of frozen-thawed ovarian cortex in sheep. Hum Reprod 14:2149–2154
66. Baird DT, Webb R, Campbell BK et al (1999) Long-term ovarian function in sheep after ovariectomy and transplantation of autografts stored at −196 °C. Endocrinology 140:462–471
67. Zhang Z, Wang ZX, Liu S (2004) Pore size, tissue ingrowth, and endothelialization of small-diameter microporous polyurethane vascular prostheses. Biomaterials 25:177–187
68. Bergmann NM, West JL (2008) Histogenesis in three-dimensional scaffolds. In: Atala A, Lanza R, Thomson JA et al (eds) Principles of regenerative medicine. Academic, Burlington, pp 686–703
69. Shi H, Han C, Mao Z et al (2008) Enhanced angiogenesis in porous collagen-chitosan scaffolds loaded with angiogenin. Tissue Eng A 14:1775–1785

70. Peters A, Baruch Y, Weisbuch F et al (2003) Enhancing the vascularization of three-dimensional porous alginate by incorporating controlled release basic fibroblast growth factor microspheres. J Biomed Mater Res A 65:489–497
71. Tanihara M, Suzuki Y, Yamamoto E et al (2001) Sustained release of basic fibroblast growth factor and angiogenesis in a novel covalently crosslinked gel of heparin and alginate. J Biomed Mater Res 56:216–221
72. Chen RR, Silva EA, Yuen WW et al (2007) Spatio-temporal VEGF and PDGF delivery patterns blood vessel formation and maturation. Pharm Res 24:258–264
73. Gigli I, Cushman RA, Wahl CM et al (2005) Evidence for a role for anti-Mullerian hormone in the suppression of follicle activation in mouse ovaries and bovine ovarian cortex grafted beneath the chick chorioallantoic membrane. Mol Reprod Dev 71:480–488
74. Camboni A, Martinez-Madrid B, Dolmans MM et al (2008) Autotransplantation of frozen-thawed ovarian tissue in a young woman: ultrastructure and viability of grafted tissue. Fertil Steril 90:1215–1218
75. Keros V, Xella S, Hultenby K et al (2009) Vitrification versus controlled-rate freezing in cryopreservation of human ovarian tissue. Hum Reprod 24:1670–1683
76. Nisolle M, Casanas-Roux F, Qu J et al (2000) Histologic and ultrastructural evaluation of fresh and frozen-thawed human ovarian xenografts in nude mice. Fertil Steril 74:122–129
77. Nottola SA, Camboni A, Van Langendonckt A et al (2008) Cryopreservation and xenotransplantation of human ovarian tissue: an ultrastructural study. Fertil Steril 90:23–32
78. Laschke MW, Menger MD, Vollmar B (2002) Ovariectomy improves neovascularisation and microcirculation of freely transplanted ovarian follicles. J Endocrinol 172:535–544
79. Amorim CA, Gonçalves PB, Figueiredo JR (2003) Cryopreservation of oocytes from pre-antral follicles. Hum Reprod Update 9:119–129

MIX
Papier aus verantwortungsvollen Quellen
Paper from responsible sources
FSC® C105338
www.fsc.org

If you have any concerns about our products,
you can contact us on
ProductSafety@springernature.com

In case Publisher is established outside the EU,
the EU authorized representative is:
Springer Nature Customer Service Center GmbH
Europaplatz 3, 69115 Heidelberg, Germany

Printed by Libri Plureos GmbH
in Hamburg, Germany